THE BOOK OF
NATURAL HAIR QUESTIONS & ANSWERS
FROM A STYLIST'S PERSPECTIVE

by Yesenia Hernandez

I0447380

outskirtspress
DENVER, COLORADO

Acknowledgments

I would like to thank and acknowledge my daughter Kayla, my mother, my aunt (Miriam Aneses), and everyone I may have forgotten that are locked behind the doors in my mind.

Ms. Sophia Jones, I learned a great deal working in your salon over the years. You did it all and made it look easy. I guess the greats always do. THANK YOU!

Author's Info

My love for hair began when I was a child. I was the only one in my home that had curly hair and I felt like the black sheep of the family, but due to the love of my mother I found my hair could do more than my straight-haired female relatives' hair could achieve. I could twist it, braid it, curl it, and even wear it straight. My mother, who is of Latin descent, always made me feel comfortable with who I am and how I looked. As a young adult, she encouraged me to enroll in cosmetology school and embrace my destiny to help and guide one curly beauty at a time.

When I graduated from cosmetology school I worked for as many different salons as I could. I wanted to learn as much as possible about all hair textures, and nothing beat on-the-job training. At one point, I worked for various salons at one time, many for little to no pay just to get my experience. I crammed in my brain what all of them had to offer, and when it was time to take my state board exams, I was confident I was going to pass, and when I did I was overjoyed.

The first year with my licenses I attended as many professional hair shows as I could and took as many classes that I could find. Little by little I taught myself, with the help of a few individuals in the hair industry, what natural hair could *really* achieve and never looked back to doing chemicals again.

Why a book on natural hair questions & answers?

I have worked full-time as a hairstylist for twelve years, but I have worked in the hair industry for twenty. After many years working for different salons and learning various techniques on all hair textures, I chose to go out on my own and work for myself. As the owner of SenKay Natural Hair Studio in Charlotte, North Carolina, I found many naturals wanted real answers about their hair questions and concerns. They were not asking your typical styling questions, nor did they want an answer that was full of fluff. These women wanted to understand what the stylist knew. After all, many of them have not seen their natural texture since they were a child; and some were mothers who adopted children from other countries with hair completely different from their own.

I felt it was imperative to help as many women as I could . . . until I had calls coming in from men who had hair concerns for their young children. I put the most frequently asked questions people asked me in a book. Some questions were asked by newcomers of natural hair while others are from seasoned vets. Either way, I have put all questions in laymen's terms so you can have a better understanding of all hair textures. I have addressed 100 percent naturals, locks (aka dreadlocks), and styling tools because without these little helpers some styles could not be achieved. My goal is for you to understand and arm you with the correct information about your hair so you feel comfortable in the decisions you make.

TABLE OF CONTENTS

Chapters

Chapter 1

100 PERCENT NATURAL: GENERAL INFORMATION

This chapter is designed to help individuals understand what their hair is comprised of. This is important because when you understand what the hair can achieve you can avoid some basic hair mistakes that can damage the mane. It is essential to grasp that all hair is not created equal, and there is more than just the basic straight, wavy, curly, and tightly coiled hair we came to learn and love. Other factors such as illness, diet, and lifestyle have a huge impact as well. We cannot forget about hair being normal, oily, dry, and damaged, or a combination of these things because they also give the hair its structure and strength.

What is natural hair?

Hair that has not been altered by chemicals would be considered natural despite hair pattern and texture. These chemicals include straighteners, perms, curl enhancers, and color. Technically, anyone without a chemical including color has natural hair, but many who have a natural mane will use color to enhance or change their looks.

Here are a few examples:

- Covering gray.
- Enhancing their natural hair tones.
- Completely changing their natural color for fashion reasons.

What are the benefits of going natural?

- Hair is less dry due to chemical use.
- On average, less money is spent on products if hair is maintained properly.
- Less shedding from chemical use.
- Less dandruff from chemical use.
- Fuller hair depending on genetics and healthy hair practices.

Who are natural stylists?

Natural stylists are generally people who work on hair that is free of chemicals. In many states, natural stylists do not need a license to work on natural hair, but in order to work with chemicals such as color, relaxers, and curl reformers, a person must obtain their cosmetologist license. By law, a license must be displayed in a salon.

What is the life cycle of <u>normal</u> healthy hair?

A healthy hair cycle will grow for a few years, rest for a few months, shed, and then regrow. All hair strands on your head will be in different growth cycles. This is why when you brush your mane all the hair does not come out at once unless illness is present. If you believe your hair is growing slower or has stopped growing, I suggest seeking a physician's advice. The three stages of a normal hair cycle are called anagen, catagen, and telogen:

- **Anagen**—The growth phase of hair. You may see your hair flourish in this stage.
- **Catagen**—Transitional phase. The end of the growth phase and the beginning of the resting phase.
- **Telogen**—The shedding or resting phase.

Will it be difficult to manage my hair once I am natural?

When you understand the needs of your hair and use the correct products designed for your hair you will find managing your own hair will be a breeze, but like anything else, *practice* makes perfect.

What are the different types of natural hair patterns?

Many cosmetology schools teach hair has four major textures: *straight, wavy, curly,* and *extremely curly.* A person can hold two or three different hair patterns on their head, but as a licensed cosmetologist, I have found wavy patterns come in the basic four but do have numerous subcategories. Andre Walker, Oprah's hairstylist, reviews categories and subcategories in his book *Andre Talks Hair!* Another individual, Lorraine Massey, also has her views on curl patterns, which includes curls that have a particular spring pattern. But one thing that must be addressed is the hair's overall health, such as, dry, oily, normal, a combination of the above, and damaged.

For example, if a person has straight hair and it is oily, it will not react to a product or style the same way as a person with dry or normal hair. I simply state this because hair texture is one thing and the overall health is another. When you analyze what they both bring to the hair table, you may be looking at product purchases in a different light. I always inform my clients if you buy products that are designed for oily, dry, normal, or a combination, or damaged hair, you can rarely go wrong.

What is curl definition?

It is the depth of the wave or spiral in the hair. If the hair is straight you will not see curl definition.

Why do some individuals' curls look better after they have blown their hair straight?

I believe the general theory is simple. When healthy hair is blown out properly, the cuticle of the hair strands lay flat, giving the hair a smooth appearance. When the hair is shampooed, the cuticles are not as rough because of the blowout, and depending on the hair texture, the hair will lack frizz after the first shampoo, but over time, the frizz will reappear. If too much heat is used during the blowout, then heat damage can occur and the cuticles of the hair can become ruined.

Does natural hair shine?

The straighter the hair the more noticeable the shine will be because light reflects better from a straighter surface than a curved one. When my curly clients request their hair to be blown straight, many are surprised of the shine their hair gives off because they do not see that same shine when their hair is curly. However, just because you do not see the shine as well when the hair is curly does not mean your hair is not healthy.[1]

How do individuals receive their hair pattern?

Hair is genetic, like the color of our eyes. It comes from the combination of our parents' DNA.[2]

Can our natural hair pattern be changed?

In short, no, it cannot. Changing a person's natural hair pattern can only be done with the use of chemicals. Most healthy individuals have one-fourth to one-half inch of new hair growth a month. This means the new growth that grows must be chemically treated to match what has already been processed, resulting in an ongoing dependence of chemicals.

Can heat alter our natural curl pattern?

Yes. If hair is exposed to high temperatures frequently or over prolonged periods, the natural curl pattern can relax, but do not confuse this with high heat damage, which can happen the first time you use heat. Usually, heat-damaged hair will be lifeless and have little or no shine, and sometimes leave a gray cast on the hair.

If hair is naturally straight you may see the heat damage better at the ends of the hair because they will become frayed. If you look under a microscope you may see *split ends*.

How do I deal with the many different curl patterns in my hair?

As a stylist and a person with many different patterns in my own hair, I find using organic shampoos with natural ingredients work best. I have also found using organic shampoos while transitioning can cut back on the tangling process because these shampoos do not have synthetic ingredients in them that can strip the hair of its natural moisture. Many true natural and organic shampoos can be found in health food stores.

What is hair texture?

Hair texture is the hair strands' thickness. Texture varies with each individual and can be different in separate areas on the same head. It can be described as smooth or rough. Texture can vary from:

- **Coarse:** Coarse hair is stronger, has the largest thickness, and can be harder to chemically process, be resistant to hair coloring, perming, and straightening.

- **Medium:** Medium texture or middle-range of thickness possesses no special considerations regarding chemical services.

- **Fine:** Fine hair or the smallest range diameter is easily processed and can be damaged from chemical exposure.

What is hair density?

The amount of hair a person has on their head per square inch is considered their density.

What is hair porosity?

It is the ability of the hair to absorb water. If the hair has high porosity levels, the hair can readily accept chemicals and cause permanent damage. It can also take more time to dry a person's hair if they have high porosities. If the hair has low porosity, it can take chemicals longer to penetrate in the hair strands.

Stylist Note:

Density can dictate how a person may wear their hair. If hair is sparse in any area of the head, it may be hard to achieve fullness and body in a hairstyle.

The porosity test is to help an individual understand how readily the hair strands absorb water and hair chemicals.

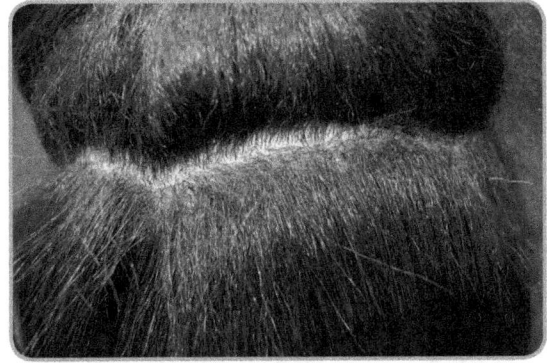

This photo is a good example of how some individuals have dense (a lot) hair. If you look close, you can see more than one hair growing from some of the hair follicles.

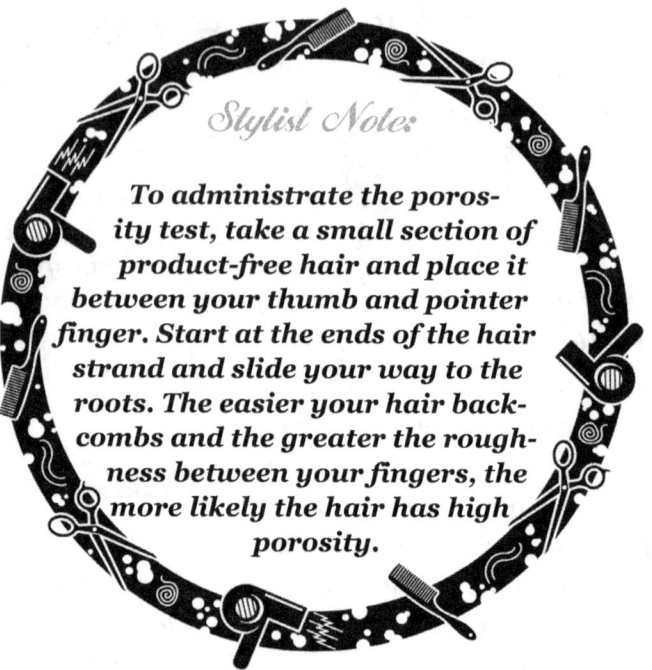

Stylist Note:

To administrate the porosity test, take a small section of product-free hair and place it between your thumb and pointer finger. Start at the ends of the hair strand and slide your way to the roots. The easier your hair backcombs and the greater the roughness between your fingers, the more likely the hair has high porosity.

What is hair elasticity?

The hair's ability to stretch and return to its original size without breaking is considered elasticity. If the elasticity is gone from the hair it will have a higher chance of breakage. Some textures can stretch up to 50 percent when wet so be cautious when combing wet hair.

What are split ends?

Split ends occur when the hair ends split from the bottom. If not cut, the split hair can work its way to the root and leave the hair lifeless, without body. It can happen from excessive styling, chemical services, not having regular trims, and brushing and/or combing roughly. Spit ends cannot be fixed, but you may slow down the process with a conditioning treatment. Overall, the best way to stop them running up the hair shaft is to cut them off.

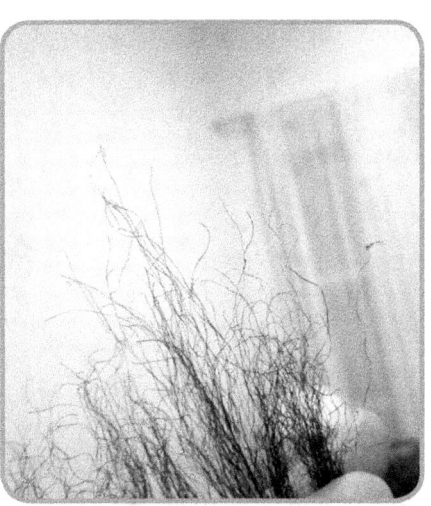

What is the best way to fix damaged hair?

Split ends and hair knots can occur on any hair texture. This can arise when hair is styled with high heat, damaged styling tools, lack of hair trims and/or rough styling to name a few.

Cut it off. This is not the answer many want to hear, but it is the best option. If the hair is damaged that means styling options are limited and it is a matter of time before the hair will split up the shaft and/or break. Some individuals may want to grow their hair out, but the truth is this can backfire and take much longer than one may expect. Damaged hair will pull moisture from the healthy hair, leaving it vulnerable to dryness, breakage, and/or split ends that will eventually travel up the hair shaft.[3]

What is hair shrinkage?

Hair shrinkage is the percentage of hair that draws up when wet or when humidity comes in contact with the hair. The tighter the curl pattern, the more shrinkage someone may have; the looser the curl pattern, the less likely the hair will draw up.

Why do some curls grow out and not long?

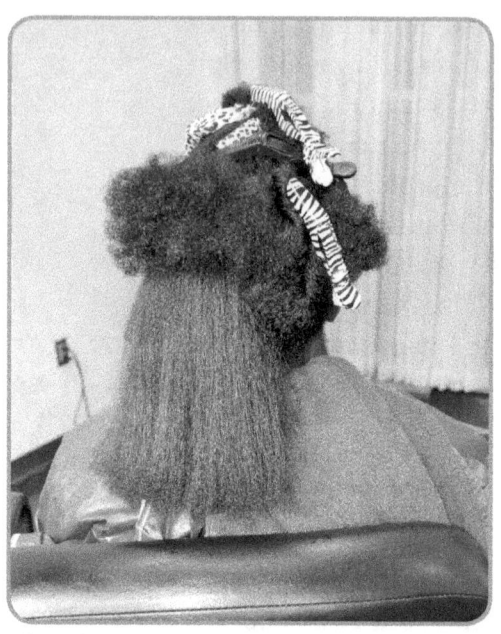

This photo is a great example of how natural curly hair can stretch when straighten.

Curls have a spiral to them whereas straight hair does not. When curly hair grows, it lays on top of each other to create height and volume due to the spirals. The tighter the curl, the more likely the hair will grow up and out and not down. This is why some curly-haired women feel their hair is not getting longer but bigger. If the curl is stretched, they will see it is longer than they expected.

If women with tightly curly hair would like more length, they have a few options:

- Blow-dry the hair, but be sure not to make the hair bone-straight.
- Cornrow, two-strand twists, flat twists, or individual plait the hair and let it dry. When you take out the style the hair will be stretched.
- Roller set the hair to elongate the hair.

What is a length check?

Very curly hair can draw-up to a tight curl and not show true hair length. Blowing the hair straight or just pulling the curl down can check the length of the hair to see how long it has grown over an extended period of time.

What is hair plateau?

Hair plateaus refer to any period of time when the hair stops growing. Do not confuse hair plateau with the normal growth cycle of hair. As a stylist, I find plateau has more to do with the care of hair than anything else. When a person uses the correct products and styling options, their hair will grow. It is when the wrong products or chemicals are used the hair will plateau. When the correct care is implemented, the hair will grow.

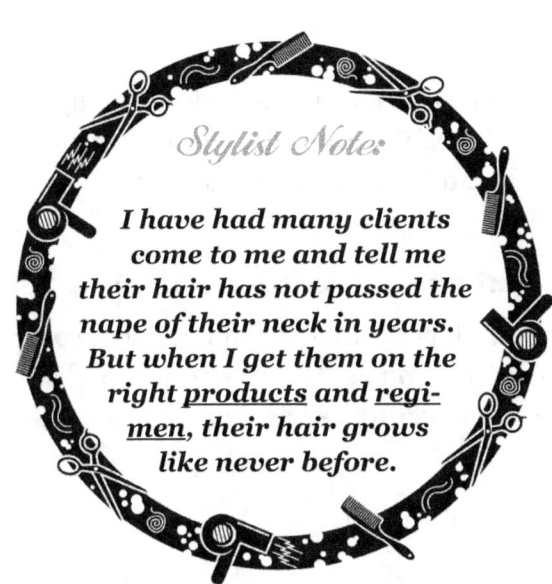

Stylist Note:

I have had many clients come to me and tell me their hair has not passed the nape of their neck in years. But when I get them on the right __products__ and __regimen__, their hair grows like never before.

Why will my hair not grow?

When the hair is not in its normal growth cycle it may lead to slow growth or shedding. Other causes can contribute to this issue as well. If the reasons below do not fit into your concerns you may want to consult with a medical doctor.

Here are some reasons:

- Unhealthy lifestyle: e.g., poor diet, smoking, drugs, etc.
- Damage to the hair follicles from chemical use or head trauma.
- Longer shedding cycles (telogen) and slower growth cycles (anagen).
- Hair is breaking from extreme heat use (blow-dryer, flat irons, etc.) and styling.

What is alopecia?

Alopecia means hair loss and can be located anywhere there is hair. Alopecia can be caused by illness, medication, taut hairstyling, and trauma from a head injury.

What is Centrifugal Cicatricial Alopecia (CCCA)?

It is a type of alopecia that is found almost completely in African American women. It is progressive and causes scaring. At the moment, little is known about CCCA.[4]

What is traction alopecia?

Traction alopecia is caused when hair is pulled too tight and the hair follicle releases the hair strand, resulting in hair loss.[5]

What is dermatitis?

Dermatitis is a general term that describes inflammation of the skin. Though it may be itchy, flaky, and sometimes uncomfortable, it is not life-threatening. Depending on the severity of symptoms, treatments can vary from over-the-counter remedies to a doctor's prescriptions.

What is pityriasis, also known as dandruff?

Pityriasis is the condition where scales usually appear on the scalp, and if gone untreated can lead to hair loss. It is best not to guess a treatment for yourself because dandruff may signal an underlining health issue. In the end, a doctor's advice may save time, money, hair loss, and correct a health issue you may have.

Why is my scalp dry and flaky?

There are multiple reasons for a dry and flaky scalp. Here are a few scenarios:

- Lack of water in the body (dehydration).
- Shampoos and other products too harsh for your hair and skin type.
- Medical conditions such as diabetes and dermatitis, just to name two.
- Environmental: Such as cold weather, air-conditioning, recycled air (airplanes and offices).

- Diet: Too much junk food, sugary sweets, and processed foods.

What can I do for an itchy scalp?

If your scalp is extremely itchy, go down the itchy checklist. If you cannot correct this problem on your own, you may want to seek a doctor's advice:

- Are you putting too many products on your hair? If so, cut back or stop. Some individuals will take one to two months to see an improvement.
- Is the scalp producing enough of its own oil? If not, you may want a dermatologist's opinion. They can help by prescribing certain medications and shampoos or teach you how to change your hair routine. It may be as simple as changing your diet.
- Are you shampooing too frequently or too little? If you are shampooing too little, you may have too much buildup. If you are shampooing too frequently, you may want to cut back because the shampoo can be drying the scalp and the oil glands do not have enough time to produce enough sebum (oil) to combat dryness.
- Are you rinsing your hair properly after shampooing and conditioning? If the product is left on the scalp it can cause irritation. Properly rinsing can avoid product buildup.
- Do you drink enough water? Dehydration can cause dry skin because the body is comprised of 60 percent water, the bones 22 percent water, and the blood 92 percent water. Water is essential to the body.

Without it, humans can only live seven days or less.[10]

- Are you on any medications? Depending on the medication it can cause a multitude of issues. The best thing to do before taking any medication is to speak to a doctor, read the insert that may come in the box, ask the pharmacist questions, or check medical Web sites for the drawbacks a drug may have on the human body.

- Do you use illegal drugs? You never know what they put in street drugs. They are not made for health benefits. Stop!

Should I use oil on my scalp?

A healthy normal scalp produces its own oil called sebum. If an outside source of oil is used, it sends a signal to your sebaceous (oil) glands to stop creating its natural oil for your scalp. Many doctors have agreed oiling the scalp is not healthy and can clog your pores. I suggest not using oils on the scalp. If the problem of dry, flaky scalp persists, seek the help of a physician, nutritionist, or both, because taking matters into your own hands may cause the condition to worsen.

Can scratching the scalp cause irritation?

Some individuals scratch their scalp with a comb or their fingernails. This is to relieve an itch or lift white flakes (dandruff) from the scalp. I suggest you do not use your fingernails but instead, use a comb and use it with caution. If you scratch too vigorously you can cause cuts, bleeding, or hair loss. If you feel you have to scratch your scalp, do it with caution and be gentle to avoid irritation.

Does natural hair require upkeep and trims?

Yes, it does. All hair, with the exception of locks, should be trimmed in order for the ends not to split and break. Natural hair may not need to be trimmed as often as chemically treated hair because it contains no chemicals to speed up the hairs' natural breakdown process, but if harsh brushing and combing take place, you may need to trim earlier. It is also important to shampoo and condition for a clean scalp and hair. Proper maintenance will ensure healthy growing hair no matter the texture.

How often should natural hair be cut/trimmed?

To keep hair healthy and depending on hair texture, I suggest every six, eight, or eleven weeks.

My suggestions are:

- **Six weeks** for the person who likes to style their hair often, especially with heat and uses color. I find some of my clients love to style often and do not always use the best methods at home. This may be fun to do, but in the end, it puts stress on the ends of your mane much quicker than normal.
- **Eight weeks** is great for the person who does not pull and tug on the hair too often but does style every once in a while. Less stress on the hair equals better ends and less breakage.
- **Eleven weeks** is recommended for the healthy hair

person. Many tightly coiled hair people do not fall into the eleven-week category because the natural hair oils (sebum) can get caught in the coils of curly hair and may not reach the ends of the strand. The result can be dry, brittle hair ends, but there are exceptions to every rule.

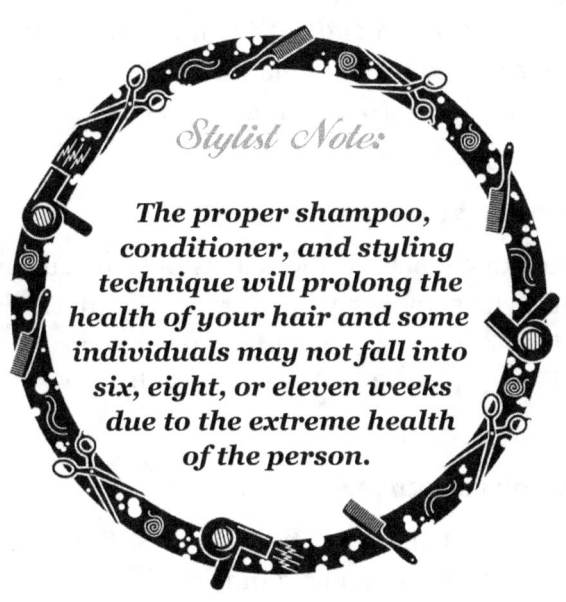

Stylist Note:

The proper shampoo, conditioner, and styling technique will prolong the health of your hair and some individuals may not fall into six, eight, or eleven weeks due to the extreme health of the person.

How do I know when I need a trim versus a cut?

Normally, a trim is anywhere from one-fourth of an inch to one-half of an inch. A cut is normally more than three-fourths of an inch and up. The longer you go without a trim, the more you may need a cut. Another great indication it is time to trim/cut is the **slide test**. The slide test can be performed on both wet and dry hair because both ways will tell a slightly different story. My preference is on dry, product-free hair that has not been flat ironed.

Performing the test

Hold a piece of your hair in between your pointer finger and thumb. Start at the root and slide down the hair shaft slowly. If you need a trim, you should feel a change in texture as you get to the ends of the hair. Some individuals will notice they may need to cut more hair in certain areas because of the extra stress that area has undergone.

Should curls be cut wet or dry?

Many individuals believe the hair should be cut one way, but great stylists know hair texture, curl patterns, and the method the stylist was trained to cut can play a big part in how the hair will be cut and the end result.

Can I razor cut curls?

I do not recommend razor cutting curls. Razor cutting in general takes skill and understanding of how the razor cuts the hair. Razors taper the ends of the hair which can cause the ends to fray.[6]

Why does my hair have more definition after I have a haircut?

Curls need moisture because hair sebum (oil) can get caught in the coils. Think of a straw that is straight and one that has twist and whirls. The straight straw will have no problem with water sliding up the straw; on the other hand, if you drink from the straw that has the bends and curves it will take longer for the water to reach the ends. Curls cause curly hair to have a lack of natural oil at the ends and cause dry, brittle hair. When you cut the dry ends off, it allows the hair to grab moisture from the air and grow healthier.[7]

Can pregnancy affect my curl pattern?

Yes, it can. Women can go through many hormonal changes when pregnant. These hormones can play a huge part in a female's mood, her skin, and hair. Some women will experience hair loss while others may experience rapid hair growth. My own personal experience and that of my clients has taught me diet is a huge key factor as well. Women who ate fruits, vegetables, nuts, and seeds closer to their natural state had a better chance of having a healthier mane. They also (myself included) had less hair shedding.

Below is a sample of what I eat in a day. You can adapt it to your liking, but make it healthy!

Semiraw Menu	Breakfast	Lunch	Dinner	Snack 1	Snack 2
Sunday	Oatmeal w/1 banana, ground flax seeds & hemp seeds, cranberries	Sprouted quinoa salad w/raw veggies of your choice & lemon juice as your dressing	Avocado, corn and tomato salad with a side of black rice & miso soup	Hummus & fresh raw veggies; broccoli, carrots, cauliflower & green beans	Fresh fruit salad; fruit of your choice. Minimum of 4 fruits

Will menopause affect my hair?

No two women are alike so menopause will affect each person differently. Diet, lifestyle, medication, family history, and hormones can play a major part in how menopause will affect your body, skin, and hair. I stress to my clients a physician's expertise would be best.

How can I get my hair to grow faster?

On average, healthy hair can grow up to a one-half inch a month. Some individuals may have more or less hair growth because of their lifestyle and diet. I can tell you from first-hand experience and as a vegan, my diet consists of fresh fruits and vegetables, as well as some form of exercise, whether it is running, playing with my daughter, biking, or just speed cleaning my house. Moving is the key. On the other hand, if you have many illnesses and take medication, the probability of having quicker hair growth is lessened. Another key component to healthy hair growth is a clean scalp. If the scalp is covered with heavy oils and dirt, it clogs the follicles hair grows from.

What is a label ninja/label savvy?

These are individuals who can read a product label and understand the majority of the ingredients on the label. If you are a label ninja/label savvy you will not fall into the **_beautiful package trap_**—*the package looks great but what is inside is awful.*

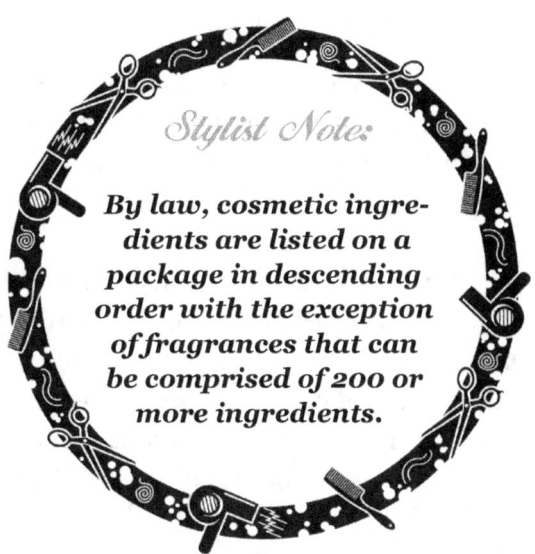

Stylist Note:

By law, cosmetic ingredients are listed on a package in descending order with the exception of fragrances that can be comprised of 200 or more ingredients.

Are consultations important before receiving a hair service?

Consultations are a great way to disclose any hair fears. To get the most out of your consultation, be sure to go in with questions and pictures of what you are trying to achieve. Remember, a picture is worth a thousand words so choose photos of what you are trying to achieve, and if your favorite hairstyle happens to be in a dish soap advertisement, then bring that picture with you so your stylist understands what you are trying to achieve.

Stylist Note:

Some stylists will charge for consultations because they are well establish and highly sought after, and time is of great importance to them.

How will swimming affect my hair?

This depends on how often you swim, where you swim, and your hair texture. The three major swimming areas are fresh water, salt water, and chemically treated water such as pools.

Fresh water rarely will have a negative effect on the hair. Normally, the hair will feel softer and the curls may have more definition, while straight hair may have more sheen. This is due to the lack of chemicals and environmental pollutants. When shampooing at home, some individuals will boil water, allow it to cool, and use it for their last rinse.

Salt water can be very rough on anyone's hair, especially if it is color treated, dry, or damaged because the salt in the water can strip hair color. It can make any texture rough and tangled. This is a great example of salt stripping the natural oils from the hair. The more you swim in salt water, the drier it may make your mane. So be sure to condition the hair often.

Chemically treated water can help or hinder the hair. If the water is chemically treated with a softening agent it may help the hair by removing impurities from the water that can strip the mane of its natural oils. On the other hand, some chemically treated water, such as pool water, may have too many chemicals in the water and strip the hair of its natural oils, causing the hair to frizz. I have also witnessed some individuals' hair turn green from the strong chemicals that are used to kill bacteria that may proliferate in swimming pools.

Who are shop hoppers/stylist hoppers?

Shop hoppers/stylist hoppers are individuals who do not stay with one salon/stylist. They go from salon to salon or stylist to stylist. The drawback to being a hopper can be very costly for your hair. Different salons and stylists use various products and techniques which can make it difficult to pinpoint what works best for your hair.

Are satin and silk pillowcases easier on the hair?

Yes. Satin and silk pillowcases do not have fibers pulling on the hair as rougher fabrics do. This makes them easier on the hair. But buyers beware; satin pillowcases can be a blend of fibers of silk and polyester so be sure to read the back of the package. Normally, if the price of the pillowcase is inexpensive, that will indicate a mixed blend.[8]

Are keratin treatments natural?

Keratin hair treatments were designed to cut back styling time and add strength to the hair by adding protein. As keratin became more in demand, so did the inquiry about the ingredients. Many individuals learned protein was not the only active ingredient in the product. Formaldehyde and other agents were key components as well. The addition of formaldehyde and the other agents make keratin treatments nonnatural.[9]

Can product lines be mixed?

Many companies design their products to work in conjunction with their product line. It is best to stay within a product line for the first thirty times of use. This will help determine if that line is right for your hair. However, there are exceptions to the rules. Many times, *true natural products* can be crossed because they do not have artificial ingredients in them that will prohibit them to work with each other.

Are hair vitamins worth the investment?

My first suggestion before ingesting any type of over-the-counter pills is to consult your physician and have a blood test. Many individuals may not go to this extent because they may feel it is not worth the trouble or money, but it is. A blood test can show more than you know about your health and could help guide you to a better well-being and stronger hair. Think of it this way: if you do not take the test, you may be ingesting something your body may not need. It may be necessary to change your overall diet because taking hair vitamins and eating fast food are counterproductive. Plus, there are many added benefits when a healthier lifestyle is put into place.

Who are salon environmentalists?

A salon environmentalist is a person or group of people that demand better health conditions for themselves, their hair, and for the environment they work in. Salon environmentalists have strict guidelines for themselves.

Here are some:

- Uses products that are made with natural and/or certified organic ingredients.

- Uses products that are safe for the environment and human use.
- Uses hair tools such as handheld dryers that eliminate or lower dangerous electrical charges.
- Uses green cleaning products to clean their surroundings.
- Recycles when appropriate.

Should I receive my hair service at natural salons because my hair is natural?

I do not believe you need to go to a natural salon if you have natural hair. Perhaps you do not live by one or want a style a natural salon does not offer. Plus, not all natural stylists work in natural salons. Some may rent rooms in another salon until they can afford to buy their own place of business. It is best to go where you, the consumer, feel comfortable. If you happen to visit a traditional salon, one that uses chemicals, it is important to explain your concerns about it. You may want to call and address your concerns over the phone before making an appointment.

Chapter 2

SHAMPOOING, CONDITIONING & HAIR TREATMENTS FOR 100 PERCENT NATURALS

Let me start by saying a clean canvas (meaning the hair and scalp) is the foundation to any hairstyle, and proper hydration is essential to long lasting healthy hair. I have spoken to many individuals who are misinformed about the simple understanding of what a clean canvas can do for your hair and overall health. I know you will find this section helpful to your needs and become aware of what a clean scalp and hair can really achieve.

How is natural hair shampooed and conditioned?

There are a few different techniques depending on the hair texture, but the general rules are:

- Start at the end by combing the knots and tangles out with a wide-toothed comb or pick. Some individuals may want to apply shampoo or conditioner on the ends of the hair to minimize breakage and help the wide-toothed comb glide through the hair.

- Wet the hair thoroughly.
- Apply shampoo to the scalp and massage into the scalp, then hair. Make sure to massage with your fingertips or a massage brush designed for your hair. If you perspire heavily or your hair is dirty, shampoo as many times as needed until the hair is clean.

Stylist Note:

Hair should be wet after, not before, all hair tangles are thoroughly removed because if hair is wet prior to removing tangles, it may be extremely difficult to comb through the hair.

- Remember, overshampooing can dry the scalp and hair and cause your tresses to frizz; the general rule is two shampoos. If you have very dense hair, a shampoo brush (e.g., Marvin Shampoo Invigorator Brush) may help you clean the scalp better than your fingertips. Nails should never be used. You may also place shampoo into an applicator bottle and squeeze the shampoo directly to the scalp.
- After shampooing, be sure to rinse completely and apply conditioner, starting at the ends of your hair and work up to midshaft if you have long hair. Be sure the conditioner does not rest on the scalp because conditioners were never made for the scalp, just the hair.
- Once the conditioner is applied, take a wide-toothed

comb and start from the nape (back of the head) and comb through. Be sure to take small sections if you have thick hair. (People with excessively curly, thick hair may shampoo with their natural hair in braided ponytails, so combing the hair may not be necessary.) If you would like to leave the conditioner on for five-to-ten minutes, and then rinse, that would be a good time to give yourself a miniconditioning treatment. I would suggest using a plastic cap in the shower because the heat from the shower may help cause the conditioner to better penetrate in the shaft of the hair.

How often should a person shampoo?

Some individuals feel it is acceptable to shampoo every two weeks, but many doctors recommend shampooing a minimum of once a week. If you perspire heavily or exercise, the "once-a-week rule" is especially important. Dirt and dust can settle on the hair and scalp and cause odor, face irritations, and sometimes breathing issues.

Stylist Note:

Over the years, and during the course of many conversations, I discovered some clients who shampooed their hair less than once a month began having breathing problems. It was not long before we determined the root of the problem. Dirt and buildup from the lack of shampooing was the cause. Once a regular routine for shampooing was put in place, these clients were amazed to see a dramatic improvement in some of the health issues they had developed— difficulty breathing, acne breakouts, and itchy scalp. All cleared up over time. The reason: unwashed hair will build up dirt and other particles, such as pollen. Dirt may attract harmful bacteria, and, for the allergic person, pollen may be responsible for the breathing problem. Keep in mind the accumulated dirt and pollen are transferred to clothing and bedding, making the symptoms increasingly worse through constant exposure, resulting in chronic health problems. Once these particles are removed through regular, more frequent shampooing, the scalp can thrive and do its job: grow hair. Just shampooing your hair may also save you money you would otherwise spend on unnecessary trips to the doctor. Obviously, if the problems persist even after changing your shampooing routine, a doctor should be consulted.

Should shampoos and conditioning products be rotated?

Rotating any hair products is not necessary, especially if the products are working. The only time an individual should rotate any product is if they change their hair structure with a chemical or use heat more frequently.[2] You may also need to rotate hair products if you travel to different climates within short spans of times.

Is sleeping on wet hair damaging?

Hair is at its weakest when it is wet, but there is no evidence sleeping on wet hair causes serious damage. On occasion, I have styled my hair with two-strand twists and pat dried my hair about 90 percent and went to bed. In the morning, I had a wonderful protective style. If you like hair accessories use them with caution when hair is wet. Hair accessories can cause hair breakage when rubbing excessively.

What is hard and soft water?

Soft water contains little to no minerals and will allow the shampoo to lather. Soft water can either be chemically treated or rainwater. On the other hand, hard water can make the lathering process difficult because of the high mineral content. If your home possesses hard water, you can use a special showerhead or attach a water softener to your water tank that will minimize the minerals in your home's water supply. Lessening hard water in your home may decrease dry, brittle hair and show the vibrancy in color-treated hair.[3]

What is a clarifying shampoo?

Clarifying shampoos are designed to remove buildup from the hair and scalp. Many of them contain vinegar to cut through the buildup on the hair, which can give the hair a lifeless appearance. I do not recommend using clarifying shampoos on a daily basis because of their stripping effects. However, I do recommend using clarifying shampoos on hair that has buildup because this is its intended use.[4]

What is a hydrating shampoo?

Hydrating shampoos are nonstripping and designed to restore moisture to dry hair. They are great for curly hair, chemically treated hair, or naturally dry hair. It adds moisture to curls that desperately need it and aids in adding moisture back into hair that has been chemically stripped of its moisture.

Are shampoo and conditioner combos (also known as a 2 in1) good to use?

No. Shampoos were originally intended to clean the hair of dirt and oils and conditioners were designed to add moisture back into your mane. I find 2 in 1 cleansers do not do a thorough job of cleaning the hair. Take the time and use a shampoo, and then a conditioner. Your hair will thank you in the long run. This is especially true for women with curly to tightly coiled hair.

What is co-washing, and is it healthy?

Co-washing is also known as conditioner washing (*using conditioner in place of shampoo, which is also known as "no poo."*) The drawback to this technique is conditioners were never intended to clean the hair and scalp. Shampoos clean the scalp and hair, and conditioners add moisture back into the hair. If you find a regular shampoo is too drying, then use a hydrating or moisturizing shampoo to help combat dryness. Keep in mind conditioners do not belong on the scalp. They can cause buildup if not rinsed properly.

What is a leave-in conditioner?

Leave-in conditioners are designed for extra hydration. Some leave-ins are creams while others are sprays. I like leave-in conditioning sprays for blowing the hair straight. Many seem to infuse the hair with extra moisture, and they do not leave an oily film on the hair like some of the hair serums.

CAUTION: If you use a cream conditioner when blowing the hair straight, be sure to use a dime-size amount. If too much cream conditioner is used, the room can become smoky or product buildup can occur.

What is a vinegar rinse?

Some individuals will use vinegar in their shampoo regimen because of the harsh buildup some products may leave. This home remedy is used by many in the health community and is dispensed from a water bottle that contains one-fourth cup of apple cider vinegar and one-half cup of water. The mix is sprayed on the hair and left on for 5 minutes, then rinsed. Some people will use it to control their dandruff, but beware: vinegar promotes blood circulation in the small capillaries that can irritate the skin so if you overuse the apple cider vinegar, you can promote dry hair and speed up dandruff issues.[6]

Are conditioners important?

Yes, conditioners can help restore moisture and strengthen the hair. I say this with a warning because many individuals believe conditioners can repair the hair to its natural state, and this is not true. They are temporary and cannot repair hair that is already damaged. Conditioners are used as preventive measures. Once the hair is damaged, it would be best to cut off the damaged part so the healthy hair can grow without the interference or challenges that come with damaged hair.

Types of conditioners

- **Humectants:** Humectants are substances that promote or absorb moisture, which helps reflect light and can make the hair appear shiny.[4]
- **Instant conditioners:** Instant conditioners fall into two types of categories. The first type is shampooed out of the hair within five minutes, and the second is a "leave-in" you can style your hair with.
- **Moisturizers:** Moisturizers are normally a cream and have a ten-to-fifteen-minute leave-in time. Many of them have a stronger staying power and penetrate deeper in the hair cuticle.
- **Protein conditioners:** Read the directions on protein treatments carefully because many of them, such as the Aphogee treatments, were designed to strengthen **chemically damaged** hair because they add body to a lifeless tress. Too much protein can have the opposite effect on hair and cause it to feel dry and break.

Are deep conditioners important?

I have found in my career as a licensed cosmetologist that many individuals misuse deep conditioners. Most people use them for longer than the time requires.

Think of the hair shaft as a sink. If you run water into a sink after a few minutes the sink will overflow and water will run onto the floor. Hair is very similar in that way. Once the hair shaft is full, it does not matter if the conditioner is left overnight; the hair strand will not accept any more conditioner.

Remember, be sure to read the directions so the product you choose to use is being used correctly and your hair can achieve the maximum benefit.

Can conditioners cause buildup?

When conditioners are used incorrectly they can cause buildup, an itchy scalp, flakes, and heavy hair.

Here are some incorrect ways conditioners are used:

- Not properly rinsing conditioners out of the hair.
- Co-washing the hair.
- Using heavier conditioners than necessary for your hair texture.

Are hot oil treatments good for the hair?

I do not use hot oil treatments. Oil and water do not make a friendly mixture because they

Stylist Note:

If conditioners are left on the scalp for long periods of time, they can cause buildup and flakes. Conditioners are made for the hair, not the scalp.

separate and usually the oils will lie on top. Because of this, I see no benefit to the hair. I prefer to use cream conditioners with a heating cap. If you insist on hot oils, use them on dry, clean hair. I find when oil is placed on dry hair and a plastic cap is placed over the hair, the tresses will readily absorb the oil.

Are protein treatments good for natural healthy hair?

Protein treatments were designed for chemically damaged hair. When the hair is styled with chemicals, such as relaxers, color, etc., the hair is stripped of its natural oils and proteins. This is where the treatments come in handy because they replenish the hair's oils and stripped protein. On the other hand, many natural hair women who use protein treatments will have dry, brittle hair because of the overuse of protein.

Are fragrances and essential oils good to use?

I believe in keeping products simple, and when it comes to fragrances and oils, you may want to be careful because they do not mean the same thing.

Fragrances can be made with many different ingredients. For example, some companies may use 200 ingredients to make one fragrance, and legally, do not have to list the 200 ingredients that comprised the fragrance. They will just put "fragrance" on the label because that is what the law allows. On the other hand, essential oils are not as complicated. Usually they are made from the oils of a particular plant or flower. But beware; just because it is natural does not mean you may not be allergic to the oil. Some oils can cause itchiness and skin irritation. The best way to test essential oils for allergies is a patch test. Put a few drops in the inner part of your arm (preferably the inner elbow) and see if you have a reaction. It is best to have the reaction on the inner part of your arm than on your scalp.

What is the difference between organic and natural?

In the hair-care industry, the rules are not stated, but there have been lawmakers and certain individuals who are trying to push companies to label more honestly and clearly with their product meaning.

Why are preservatives used in products?

Preservatives are used in products to prolong the shelf life and lower the chances of bacteria growth. Many preservatives are synthetic, but as technology advances and natural hair becomes more popular, we should see more natural preservatives used in products.[5]

Here are a few examples:

- **Neem Oil**—Antifungal, antibacterial, and spermicide.[5]
- **Salt**—Draws out moisture and generates an environment uncongenial to bacteria.[5]
- **Sugar**—Inhibits bacterial growth after products have been heated.

- **Lemons**—This rich vitamin C fruit removes moisture to prevent spoilage and rotting the same way
  sugar does.[5]
- **Honey**—Because of its low moisture content, anti-
  microbial, and low pH, honey is a great stabilizer in
  microbial growth.[5]

Are homemade hair products safe to use?

I find homemade products are good to use *as long as you do
your homework.* Do not think because a product is "homemade" it is better for you. One of my clients used a "friend's"
recipe for a hair protein mask, and the only thing that hap-
pened was the egg whites were still in her hair two days
later. When she told me what the ingredients were and the
process she used, it did not take me long to figure out the egg
cooked under the dryer. So please, do your homework and
proceed with caution because some of the best hair products
on the market today started in someone's kitchen.

Chapter 3

STYLING QUESTIONS

Understanding what the different styles are and how they differ from each other can eliminate a lot of confusion and headaches when styling the hair. Knowledge is the key, and the correct terminology will get you there. Many of these terms are used in cosmetology schools and salons across the country. Some of the terms have been around for years and others will be new, but overall, the terms and questions are used to head you in the right direction when creating your style, regardless of your hair texture.

What is a wash-&-go?

Many believe a wash-&-go is simply shampooing your hair, letting it curl, and walking out the door. Despite what many may think, a wash-&-go is a wash-&-work and is not easy for any hair texture, and the hair does need to be managed in some form. Whether it is brushing out the tangles, moisturizing, or blow-drying to relive the hair from some of its moisture, it takes work to have a wash-&-go, or shall I say, wash-&-work.[1]

What is thermal styling?

Thermal styling is the use of heat. It can be in the form of a handheld blow-dryer, a curling iron, or a crimper, to name only a few.

What is wet styling?

It is manipulating the hair into a shape or styling the hair while wet and allowing the hair to dry. Finger waving and pin curls are examples of wet styling.

It is important to allow the hair to dry 100 percent for a wet set style to last. If your hair has any moisture in it or rain and humidity reaches it, your new style will revert to your natural hair state and may frizz and/or fall flat.

What is curl forming?

Curl forming may be done with chemicals, but on natural hair it can be done by thermal or wet styling. Curl forming is a way to make your natural curls a different size. Many natural individuals set their hair on different-sized rollers from their natural curl or use a curling iron to format a curl. The same can be said about straight hair.

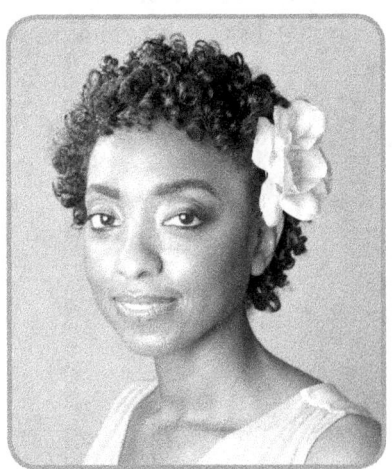

Natural textured hair can be set on perm rods, flexi rods or other types of rollers to give a frizz free curly afro.

What is the best way to comb my mane?

The hair type determines the comb-out method, but a general rule of thumb is to use a wide-toothed comb or a pick no matter what the hair texture. This ensures minimum to no breakage. Start at the ends of the hair and work your way to the scalp with gentle strokes. If the hair is tangled, a little conditioner on the ends will help the comb slide through the hair. If the hair is extremely curly, you may want to use a heavy cream conditioner, but remember, hair may stretch up to 50 percent when wet so be careful when combing.

What is backcombing?

Backcombing is also known as _teasing_ and _backbrushing_. This is a technique used to help give height and shape to hair and longevity to hairstyles. The shorter hairs are brushed down toward the scalp to create a cushion base, while hair is smoothed over the cushion base to create height.[2]

Different kinds of haircuts:

* **Big Chop (BC)**

  When an individual cuts the chemicals out of the hair, they have received the _Big Chop_ (BC). The big chop does not have to mean supershort hair or be bald.

  I had women walk into my hair studio and thought the big chop was their only choice, but this is not so. After cutting out the chemicals, they were left with two to three inches of hair, leaving them with enough hair to have a style, such as a coil-out or spiky blowout.

- **Blunt**

  Blunt cuts are also known as precision cuts or Chinese bobs. The hair is cut into one level to create a sleek one-line hairstyle.

- **Buzz/Clipper Cut**

  When hair clippers are used to cut the hair close to the scalp it is considered a buzz cut.

- **Asymmetric**

  Hair is cut shorter on one side of the head than the other.

- **Symmetrical**

  Hair is cut the same on both sides of the head.

- **Layered**

  Hair is cut into different lengths to create a waterfall effect.

What are finger combing, finger styling & finger detangling?

Using your fingers to style or rake through the hair is considered finger combing, finger styling, or finger detangling. This technique is wonderful for individuals who suffer from hair breakage.

What is finger parting?

Using your fingers and not a comb to part your hair is finger parting.

What is finger twisting?

When hair is twirled around the fingers or the fingers are used to twist the hair without the use of a hair comb.

What is finger waving?

In the 1920s and 1930s, finger waving was the rage. The S pattern waves are designed on wet hair and the only tools that were used were setting lotion, your fingers, a comb, and sometimes clips. By manipulating the comb and your fingers on wet hair, the hair would take the pattern of a wave, hence, finger waves.[3]

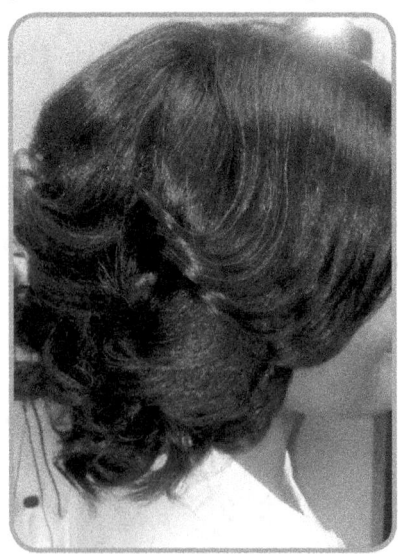

These beautiful waves were created on natural hair with the aid of a blow-dryer and flat iron. To keep this style looking crisp, be sure to pincurl the hair at night while sleeping.

What is hot waving?

Hot waving is done on dry hair and gives a similar effect as finger waving, but the tools used are combs and curling irons. To achieve a wave effect, blown-out hair is combed straight down, starting from the top of the head and working your way to the ends. Then the hair is *pinched* with the opening of the hot iron. This is done section by section to create a wave look in the hair. Be sure to let the hair cool down before touching the wave. Touching hot hair can cause the waves to fall.

What does "bumping" the ends of the hair mean?

When the hair is "bumped," it is worn straight with the hair slightly bent under at the ends.

What is a ponytail?

When the hair is secured into place with a hair tie, rubber band, or scarf, a ponytail is made. A ponytail can be placed in any area of the head.

What is a pineapple ponytail aka the unicorn?

When the hair is placed on top of the head in a loose ponytail to retain curls it is considered a pineapple ponytail (aka the unicorn).[4] Many individuals with curly hair will use this method to reduce shampooing daily.

What is plopping?

Using a towel or paper towel to remove the excess water from the hair without disturbing the natural curl is considered hair plopping. Many women perform plopping by squeezing or scrunching the hair, never rubbing the cloth through the curls because it will cause frizz.

What is hair scrunching?

Scrunching occurs when hair is gently placed in the hand and the fingers slowly open and close. It is similar to plopping without a cloth. This helps reduce frizz, maintain curls, and eliminate excess water in the hair when drying the hair with a diffuser.

How can I eliminate the frizz in my hair?

Hair is mainly constructed of hair protein called keratin, water, and lipids. If any of these three components are compromised in the hair, it can cause the hair to frizz.[8]

Here are some helpful hints to keep the frizz at bay:

- Make sure your hair is healthy. Excessively frizzy hair can be a sign of unhealthy, overly heated, dry, or processed hair.
- To eliminate frizz you want to use shampoos, conditioners, and hair products that are designed for your hair type (dry, oily, or chemically processed). Be sure to eliminate products that are alcohol-based products because they cause dryness.
- Be sure not to disrupt natural curls when squeezing the moisture out of the hair; use your hand or a fibreless towel. Example: Paper towels.
- Touch less: The less you touch your hair the better the curl will be retained.

What are the best products to use on natural hair?

(Shampoos, conditioners, creams, oils, etc.)

I like natural products that do not contain synthetic ingredients. I would also like to suggest purchasing your beauty products at a reputable health food store or salon, regardless of hair texture, because many health food stores do not carry products that contain harsh ingredients. Health stores have a reputation to uphold. Many stores do most of the work for you and rid their shelves of unfavorable products. This does not mean you walk into the store blind. Do your research before shopping any establishment and check online for product ingredients. Checking Web sites may cut down your foot traffic and save you time in the end.

Are "white hair products" OR "black hair products" just for that ethnic group?

No. Read the labels. Do not concern yourself with the picture of the person who may be on the label or in the advertisement. The ingredients tell the story of the product. It will tell whether the product works for straight, wavy, or curly hair. Also look for products that state for oily, dry, or damaged hair because they work just as well. That is what you should focus on. Sometimes it will say on the front of the bottle what hair texture/type the product is suitable for.

What is a product junky?

An individual who buys and uses a multitude of hair products on the market is considered a product junky. Many product junkies have shelves filled with products they may have used once or twice. Many times, the products they use are not for their hair texture and do not work the way they hope.[5]

What is the product graveyard?

I believe many individuals had a "graveyard" somewhere in their house at one point in time. For product junkies, usually it is under their bathroom sink with all the products that do not work on their hair texture. Instead of donating or swapping them out, they let the products collect dust and build up like dead bodies in a graveyard. If something does not work for your hair, donate it to shelters or give them to friends.[5]

What is buildup?

Buildup on the hair normally comes from placing product on top of old product. This can cause a film over the hair strands. Buildup can also form from color, such as henna, and leave the hair limp and difficult to style. Another form of buildup is dandruff buildup. This can occur when the scalp is not cleaned properly. Old flakes are left on the scalp, and new flakes form under them.

What are protective styles?

Protective styles protect the hair from the everyday heat and damage we can cause to our own hair from styling. A few good examples of protective styles are roller sets, coil-outs, two-strand twists, cornrows, and updos done with little to no product. In all, it is best not to pull and tug on the hair every day. I find protective styles are helpful and many of my clients have great success growing their hair.

What is a rod set/roller set?

The hair is set on rollers to create curls that can be large, medium, or small. You can also set the hair to create spirals which is a rod set. Roller sets give the hair body and are wonderful to transition to natural.

Different kinds of rollers:

- **Perm Rod**—Perm rods are plastic and come in many different sizes that are determined by color. They were originally designed for curly perms but have found a new function in the natural hair world for spiral sets.

- **Flexi Rods**—Flexi rods are exactly what they sound like, rods that flex. These rods also come in a range of colors that determine their size. Flexi rods give a spiral effect.

- **Curl Formers**—Curl formers are a different kind of roller that

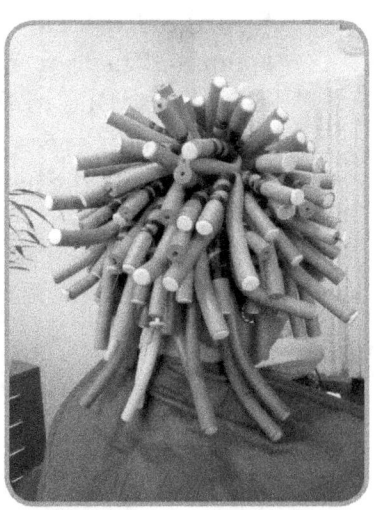

Flexi rod sets on natural hair are a great way to achieve a curly hairstyle with smooth nonfrizzy curls.

is made of soft mesh and gives the hair a spiral effect. (www.curlformers.com)

- **Straws Set**—Straws are used as a roller to create very small spirals on the hair.
- **Wrap-A-Loc**—This tool is similar to a flexi rod, but on a much-smaller scale. A person can wrap a lock around the tiny flexible strawlike roller or loose hair to make minispiral curls that resemble a straw set. (www.wrapaloc.com)
- **Velcro**—Used on dry hair only and are banned in some states to use in a salon because they cannot be sanitized but are great for home use.
- **Hot Rollers**—Hot rollers are rollers that are heated in a heated tray to make the rollers warm. The rollers are placed on dry hair and are allowed to cool down to achieve a strong curl set.[6]
- **Sponge Rollers**—Sponge rollers are made from sponges. They are normally round and can create tight curls. Due to the sponge material, I strongly suggest end papers or the satin cover rollers. This will eliminate the hair sticking to the rollers and creating frizz.

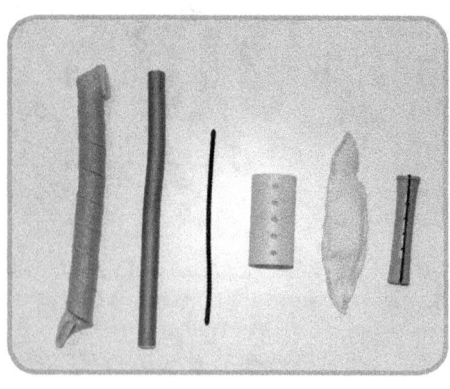

From left to right: curlformer, flexi rod, wrap-a-loc, magnetic roller, pillow top roller, perm rod.

What is a pin curl?

A pin curl can be done on dry or wet hair. The hair is curled by hand from the bottom up using some sort of a hairpin to hold it in place. This is great for someone that hates to sleep with rollers and would like to retain their curls for the next day without using excessive heat.[7]

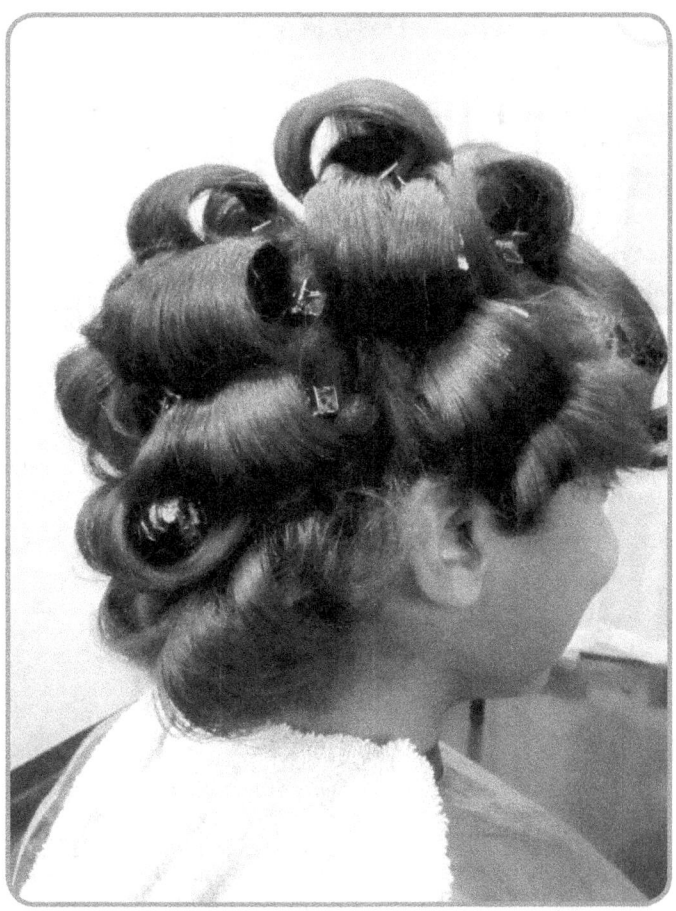

Stand-up pincurls are used to create fullness in the hair when styled. They are also a great alternative to sleeping in rollers.

What is base clipping?

Base clipping is used to create height in curls that may be heavy at the base/root of the hair. Prong clips are used in the base-clipping technique.

Two types of prongs may be used.[9]

- **Single prong**—Has one prong on it and works like a bobby pin.
- **Double prong**—Has two prongs on it and is used more frequently in the base-clipping technique because it gives the hair more height.

What is a pinup/updo?

This style pulls the hair up and off the face. A person can have medium to long hair and hold it in place with hair pins and accessories. Some updo styles are:

- **Chignon**—Can be made from a ponytail placed in a ball which can be messy or tidy and classic.
- **French twist**—A French twist can be a basic or classic hair tuck. The basic twist is tidy and sleek while the classic twist is tall and big.[10]

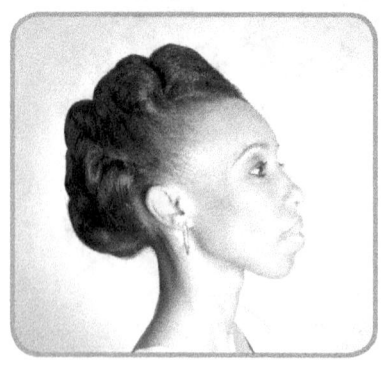

Our model, Brittney, has tight curly hair which has been blown semi straight with warm heat to elongate her curls. Next, Brittney's hair was tucked and pinned in place with bobby pins to create this elegant updo.

What is a blowout?

This is when a blow-dryer is use to dry the hair straight. Sometimes a pick on the end of the blow-dryer, a paddle brush, or a round brush is used to stretch the hair straight. Depending on the desired style, a flat iron can be used to assist in the smoothing process.

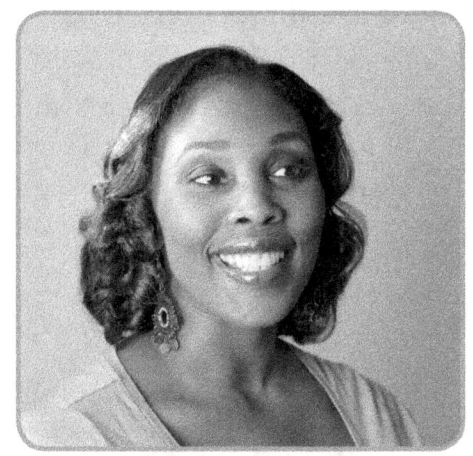

This wonderful blowout is created with a blow-dryer, denman brush and a curling iron. To keep the curls on the ends of the hair, pincurling or roller setting at night would be recommended.

Stylist Note:

If a flat iron or other heated tool is used to create a straighter style, be sure to use it only once and on the proper heat setting. Many people will continue to use a heating tool every day to keep the hairstyle as long as they can. This can cause heat damage and cause the hair to not revert back to curls when shampooed. If you are wearing curls and want the curls to last, pin curl or roller set the hair to maintain the freshness of the style. If you exercise, it would be best to place the hair in ponytails, a bun, or pin curls to keep the style fresh.

What are single twist/coils?

A single twist/coil can be created with a comb or your fingers, depending on your hair texture. When a coil is created, it will look like an elongated curl. You can make a single twist/coil in different sizes by the amount of hair you use.

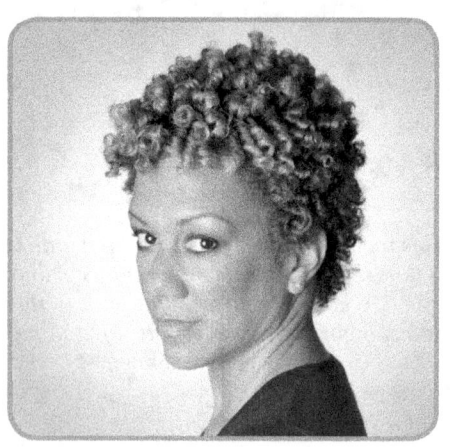

This beautiful coil out gives a frizzy afro shape, depth and style.

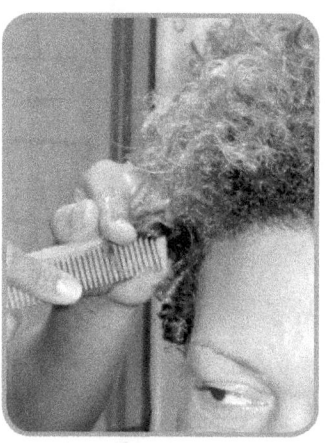

Comb coils are made with a comb and your favorite hair holding product, such as foam or a curl cream. The comb is used to coil the hair into a curl.

What is a coil out?

I love coil outs, especially on women with very curly thick hair. It shows the true beauty of what thick, excessively curly hair can do. The curls should be well defined and soft to the touch.

What is a two-strand twist aka rope braid?

A two-strand twist is two pieces of hair twisted or wrapped

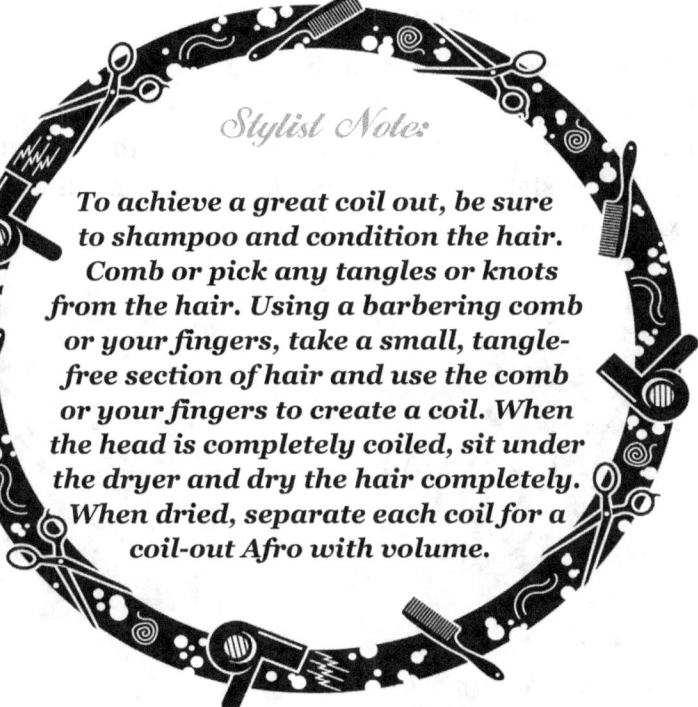

Stylist Note:

**To achieve a great coil out, be sure
to shampoo and condition the hair.
Comb or pick any tangles or knots
from the hair. Using a barbering comb
or your fingers, take a small, tangle-
free section of hair and use the comb
or your fingers to create a coil. When
the head is completely coiled, sit under
the dryer and dry the hair completely.
When dried, separate each coil for a
coil-out Afro with volume.**

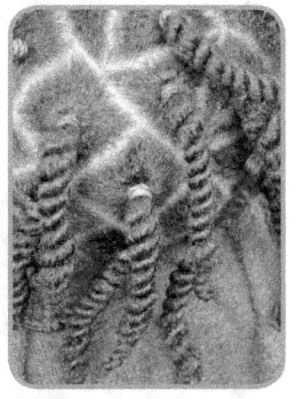

around each other to create a rope-like braid. This technique is a top protective style for many curly-haired individuals, as well as creating chignon updos for straight hair. Two-strand twists can be achieved with your natural hair or extensions.[11]

*Ponytails make a great
protective style for
children, as long as the
tension of the rubber band
does not pull the hair tight.*

What is a two-strand flat twist?

The hair is twisted flat to the head to create rows of ropelike braids. The two-strand flat twist is a method that is great for exercising and to keep you cool during the hot summer heat. This style can be achieved with your natural hair or extensions.

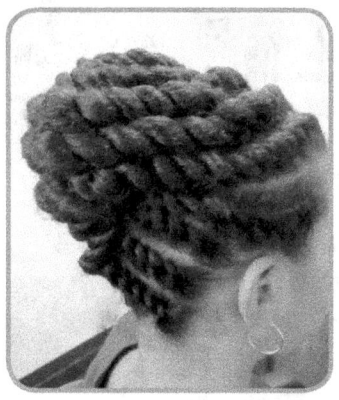

A flat twist updo can give a regal look to any natural hair do, and keep you cool during your morning workouts or on hot summer days.

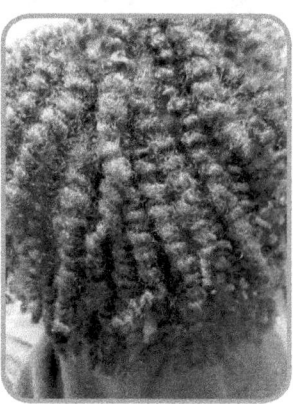

This close up of a twist out shows the beautiful pattern the hair can take when the twist are release.

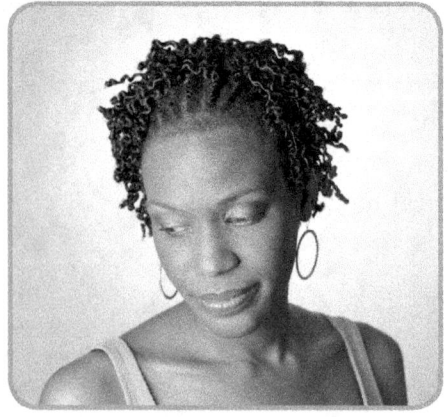

Twist outs can give your hair a wonderful textured style and a look to remember.

What is a two-strand twist-out?

A twist-out is when the hair is twisted (individually or flat to the head), completely dried, and then untwisted to form a wavelike pattern in the hair. The size of the twist can determine the size of the wave.

My twist-outs do not last long. What can I do to make my style last longer?

The hair texture can play a big part in the longevity of the style. If the hair is a straight to wavy texture, it may be better to braid the hair because braids are made with three strands and may hold better, but if the tress is damaged, any style you attempt may not last.

What is a braid?

A braid is three pieces of hair placed one over the other. It is very similar to a two-strand twist but with three pieces of hair. Braids can be done with one's natural hair or with hair extensions.

What is a fishtail braid?

The fishtail braid has the pattern that resembles the design of a fish's tail.

What are cornrows?

In the United Kingdom cornrows are also known as **track braids** or **flat braids**. This braiding technique keeps the hair flat to the scalp by picking up hair as the stylist braids.

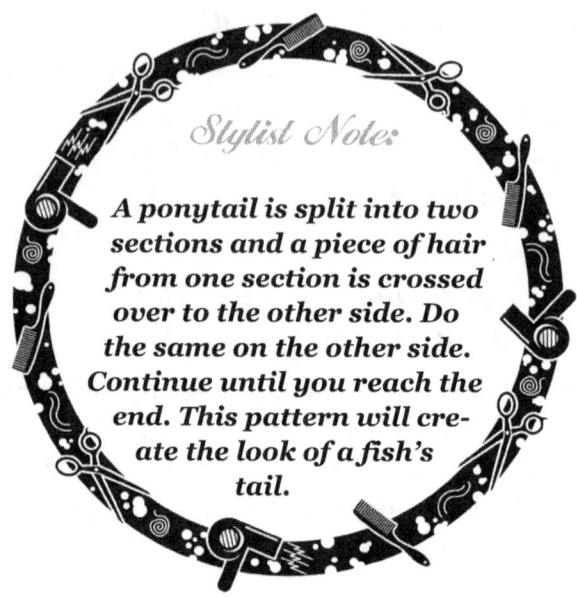

Stylist Note:

A ponytail is split into two sections and a piece of hair from one section is crossed over to the other side. Do the same on the other side. Continue until you reach the end. This pattern will create the look of a fish's tail.

Cornrow styles may be created by using a person's own hair or with extensions.[13]

What are micro-braids?

Micro-braids are done with human or synthetic hair and depending on the head size can range from 200 to 500 braids.

What is a braid-out?

The hair is braided, completely dried, and then taken out to create a wavylike texture effect on the hair.

What is an Afro puff?

An Afro puff is made when very curly hair is pulled into a

ponytail and the hair resembles a beautiful ball of cotton. Afro puffs come in many different sizes depending on the length of hair.

What are Bantu knots?

Bantu knots are also known as China bumps, Nubian knots, or cinnamon rolls, just to name a few. They are created by sections of hair (braided, twisted, or loose) wound around itself until it creates a bun.[14]

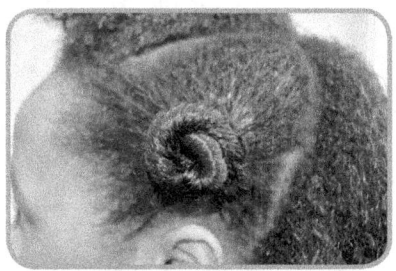

Bantu knots are used to create curly styles in the hair, or keep the hair out of the way when styling another section.

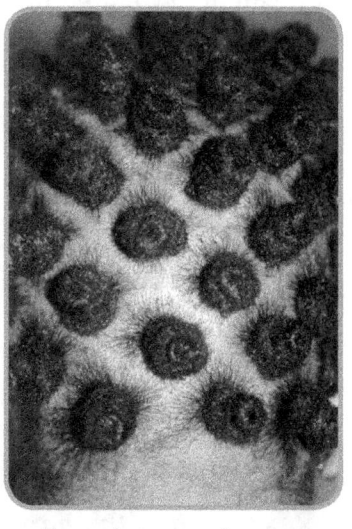

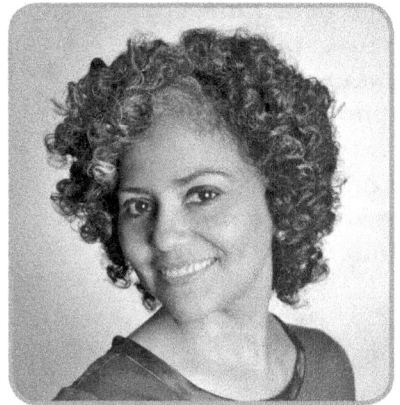

Bantu knots can be worn with locks as shown here as a style, and taken down later to give a second style to locks as crimps/curls.

Bantu knot outs are a nice way to change your natural curl pattern without rollers.

What is a Bantu knot out?

Bantu knot outs are created when dried Bantu knots are un-wound and the hair is left with a wavy pattern. The pattern is dictated by the size of the Bantu knot and hair texture.

Should I cover my hair when I sleep?

This depends completely on the individual. Some prefer to sleep without a head covering. I, for one, hate to cover my head so I use satin pillowcases, but if you feel covering your hair can help you maintain a healthy mane, then go for it.

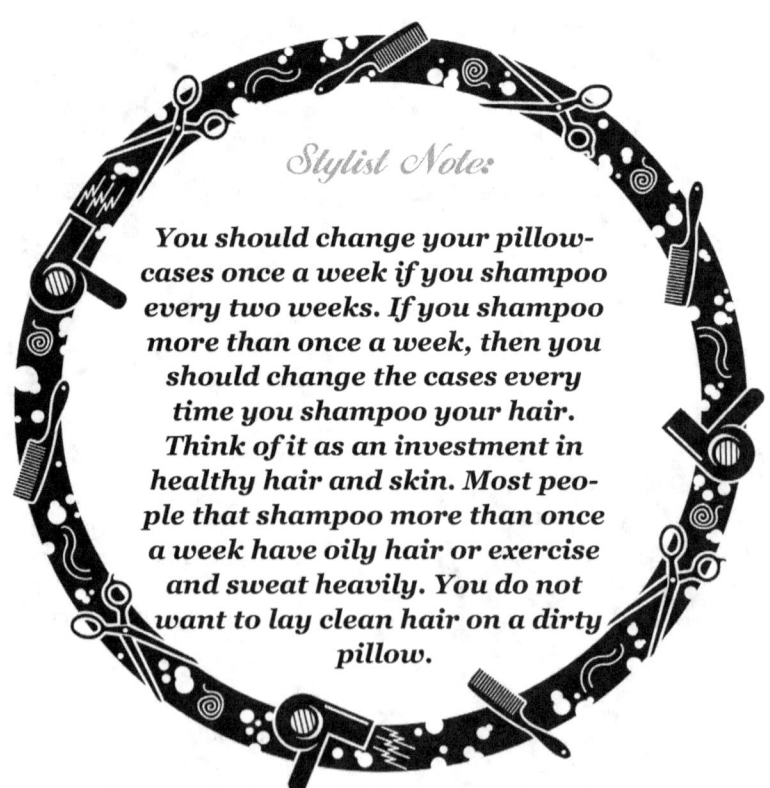

Stylist Note:

You should change your pillow-cases once a week if you shampoo every two weeks. If you shampoo more than once a week, then you should change the cases every time you shampoo your hair. Think of it as an investment in healthy hair and skin. Most people that shampoo more than once a week have oily hair or exercise and sweat heavily. You do not want to lay clean hair on a dirty pillow.

Should natural hairstylists be taught about chemicals?

Due to the lack of laws in the hair-care industry, at this time, many states do not require natural stylists to be licensed. I believe if natural stylists are required to learn about chemicals, the client will benefit, especially if the client chooses to transition out of chemicals or has scalp damage from prolonged chemical use.

How can exercising effect my hairstyle?

The style you wear and the hair texture will determine how your hair will hold up during your exercise routine.

Can constant tension disturb a person's natural curl pattern?

Yes, if the hair is constantly pulled into a ponytail, especially when wet, you may notice when the ponytail is removed certain sections of the hair will remain straight. If the ponytail is always being worn, it can cause permanent hair straightening because the hair's hydrogen bonds are broken. Hydrogen bonds make up one-third of the hair's total strength. This is the reason a physical change occurs when the hair dries from a wet set.

Do weather conditions dictate a hair routine?

Absolutely! People with curly hair may notice more of a routine swing than someone with straight hair. Have you ever noticed in warm weather how some curly girls' hair will swell? Some individuals will love the big hair look while others may not. With that being said, if you travel like I do, you may have to pack different hair products for different regions of the country, even if the season is the same because certain regions may be warmer or cooler than others and that can affect the hair just as weather can affect your skin.

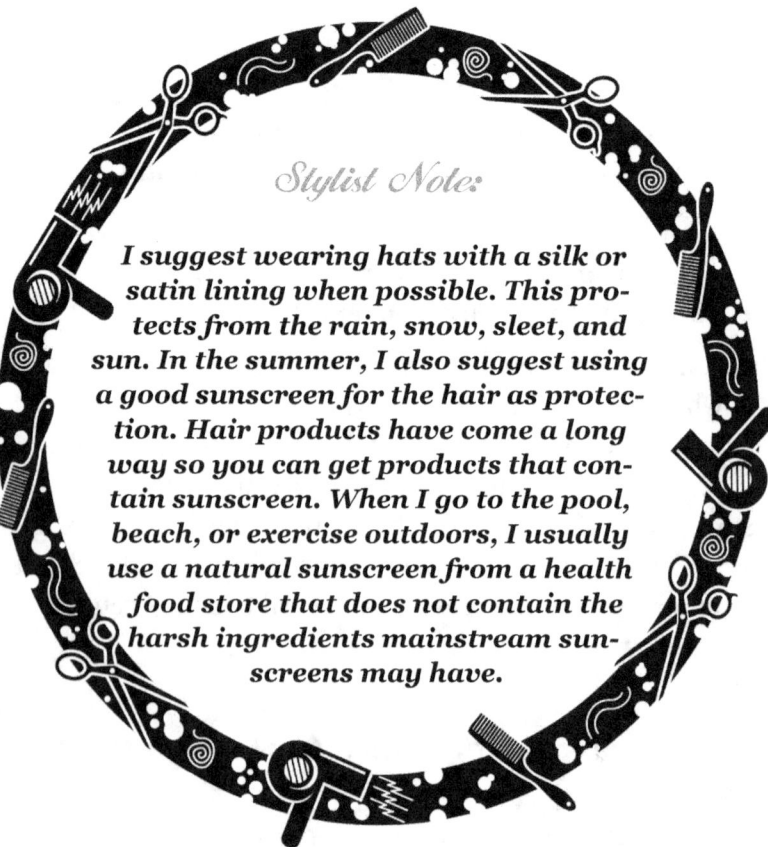

Stylist Note:

I suggest wearing hats with a silk or satin lining when possible. This protects from the rain, snow, sleet, and sun. In the summer, I also suggest using a good sunscreen for the hair as protection. Hair products have come a long way so you can get products that contain sunscreen. When I go to the pool, beach, or exercise outdoors, I usually use a natural sunscreen from a health food store that does not contain the harsh ingredients mainstream sunscreens may have.

Chapter 4

STYLING TOOLS & AID QUESTIONS

No matter what the hair type we all need some form of styling tool and aid to achieve our look. This chapter will help you understand the proper names of each tool and its function. Without these styling aids, we could not create the joys we consider part of our personality. Keep an open mind when reading this section because different stages of being natural, textures of hair, and hair lengths will require different tools to achieve their styling goals. Plus, what you may have used two years ago may not be the same tools you would use today because your hair may have changed due to pregnancy, health issues, age, or diet. No person's hair is completely the same.

What is a blow-dryer?

A blow-dryer is a handheld device that can have a variety of speeds and heat settings. Some blow-dryers come with different attachments such as a comb (also known as a pick), diffuser, or different nozzle sizes. Handheld blow-dryers have come a long way so finding one that suites your needs is a lot easier than years ago.[1]

Are blow-dryers good to use?

Blow-dryers can be helpful when used correctly. They can help define curls when a diffuser is used or help straighten the hair before the use of a flat iron, but I will warn you, be careful of the settings. A dryer that is too hot can scorch the hair, create flyaways, and lose elasticity in the hair.

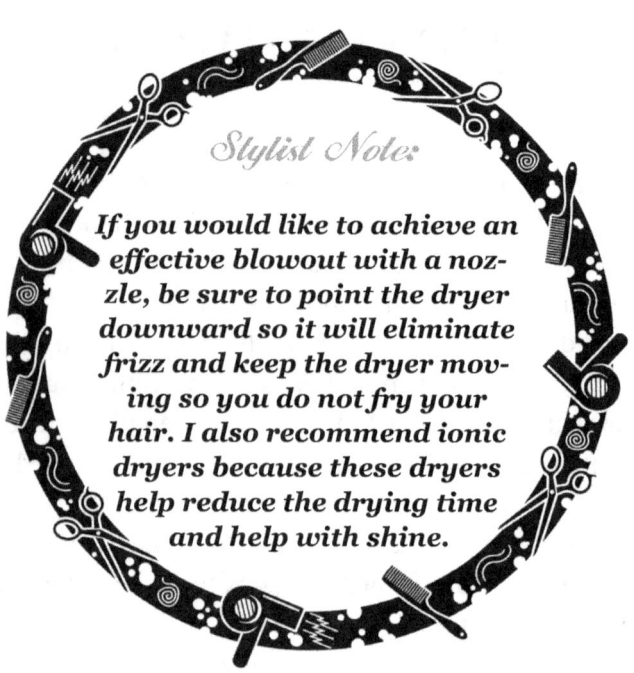

Stylist Note:

If you would like to achieve an effective blowout with a noz-zle, be sure to point the dryer downward so it will eliminate frizz and keep the dryer moving so you do not fry your hair. I also recommend ionic dryers because these dryers help reduce the drying time and help with shine.

What is a diffuser, and how is it used?

A diffuser is a tool that attaches to the end of a blow-dryer and allows the air to flow out without force. Diffusers come in all shapes and sizes. Some blow-dryers come with a diffuser in the box.[1]

What is a pick attachment on a blow-dryer?

A pick attachment is a comb that is attached to the nozzle of a handheld blow-dryer. It is used to comb the hair straight while simultaneously drying the hair. The pick attachment is often used for home use by individuals with tightly coiled hair.

What is a hooded dryer?

A hooded dryer is a device a person sits under while warm air circulates out from the holes inside the hood to dry the hair.[2]

What is a heating cap?

A heating cap looks similar to a hat that plugs into a wall socket. It is used to add moisture back into the hair without the use of forced heated air or steam. The heating cap is a great alternative for individuals that cannot use a steamer due to breathing issues.

What are flat irons and hair crimpers?

Flat irons are devices that have smooth heated plates on two sides. They may have straight plates or curved ones that are called C plates. C plate flat irons are great to add curls or give the ends of the hair a slight bend. Hair crimpers are similar to flat irons, but with one exception. Crimpers have wavy plates to create different depths of waves and crimps, whereas straight plates are used to smooth the hair straight.[1] You can find them with ceramic, titanium, or a combination of both technologies that coat the plates of the irons. I would recommend buying irons that have a temperature gauge you can control.

What is ion technology?

In the hair-care industry, ion technology creates negative ions to combat the positive ions in the hair. Negative ions help the hair to absorb moisture, which is great for dry hair and for preventing frizz and static that can cause damage. Ionic components, such as a flat iron, are a wonderful option for straightening curly hair. These components neutralize electrical charges and help the mane to lay flat and smooth. Ion technology is great for people who like to wear their hair straight but do not like chemicals to achieve the straight look.[3]

Are ceramic and titanium heat instruments good to use?

The great thing about today's hair instruments is the technology. Years ago, hair irons had to be heated in the fire or on a stove, but now we can simply plug them in and adjust the temperature that works best for our hair. Ceramic and titanium instruments are wonderful tools for the hair because they do not singe the hair like the old irons did in the 1980s. Ceramic and titanium irons have a special coating on them that will not allow the hair to stick and burn like the old irons used to do.

Are heat protectants necessary for the hair?

I have never believed oil- or cream-based products were protecting the hair, especially the ones that are made from oils and silicones. These protectants can burn the hair and cause a smoky room; plus, I never understood the concept of oil-based products protecting the hair. I have shampooed clients and the scent from heat protectant products would not shampoo out.

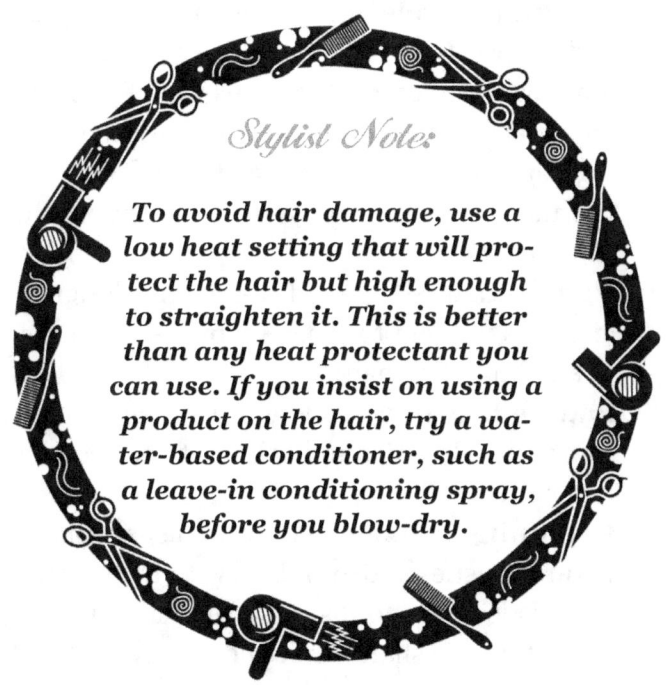

Stylist Note:

To avoid hair damage, use a low heat setting that will protect the hair but high enough to straighten it. This is better than any heat protectant you can use. If you insist on using a product on the hair, try a water-based conditioner, such as a leave-in conditioning spray, before you blow-dry.

What is a wide-toothed comb?

A wide-toothed comb has teeth that are not set close together. This will help minimize breakage and help the comb pass through the hair.[4] Wide-toothed combs come in different sizes and styles.

What is a rattail comb?

A rattail comb has a pointed handle on one end and small-to-medium teeth on the other. Many stylists use this comb to weave highlights through the hair or to create straight parts for cornrows or a roller setting.[5]

What are the different types of hairbrushes?

- **Round brushes**—They come in an array of sizes and shapes. Some brush bristles are made from nylon, boar bristles, or a combination of both. The client's hair should wrap twice around the brush for a great blowout. To create a strong curl, be sure to use the cool button on your blow-dryer to hold in the curl.
- **Vent brushes**—These brushes are designed with air vents in them to speed up blow-drying time and to add lift to fine hair.
- **Paddle brushes**—Paddle brushes are wide in design with nylon pins and ball tips to protect the scalp and hair.
- **Grooming brushes**—They are usually made with natural bristles and/or mixed with nylon. The natural bristles help to dispense the hair's natural oils down the hair shaft, while the nylon bristles stimulate the blood in the scalp.
- **Denman brushes**—Denman brushes have been around since 1938 and were made popular by Vidal Sassoon in the 1950s when he used Denman brushes to create the perfect blowout. Today, straight hair naturals use the brush to recreate the Vidal blowout,

and many curly naturals use the Denman to relieve the hair of tangles and create their straight blowout.[6]

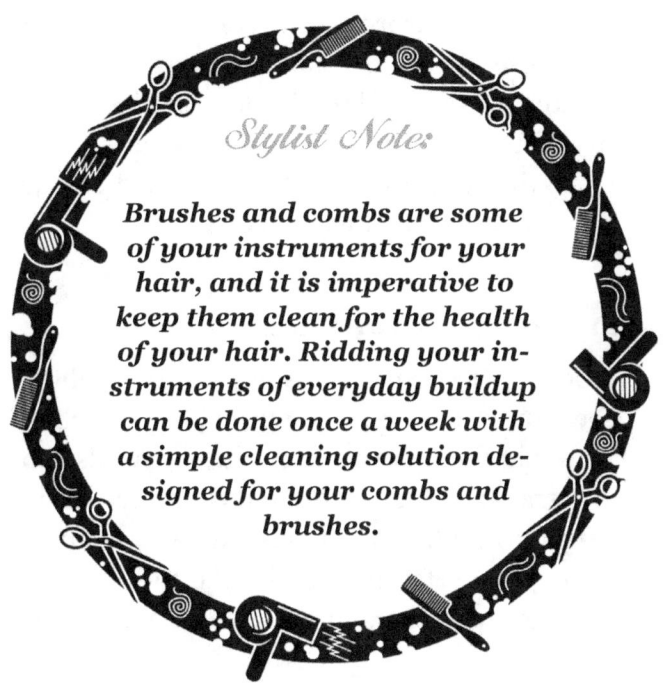

Stylist Note:

Brushes and combs are some of your instruments for your hair, and it is imperative to keep them clean for the health of your hair. Ridding your instruments of everyday buildup can be done once a week with a simple cleaning solution designed for your combs and brushes.

Cleaning steps for your combs and brushes

- Manually clean as much hair from your combs and brushes as possible.
- Place hot (not boiling) tap water in a container or fill a clean sink with enough water to submerge your combs and brushes.
- Add a cleaning solution designed for your brushes. I recommend Spic and Span for brushes and combs. You can find it in beauty supply stores such as Sally Beauty Supplies. Be sure to read the directions for

the proper water to solution ratio.

- Submerge your brushes and combs in the solution for the recommended time length.
- Remove the hairbrushs and combs from the solution and rinse them with clean fresh water.
- Lay the brushes and combs on a towel to dry or hand dry them.
- Once they are dried, place in a sealed container to protect them from dust and dirt.

What are bobby pins and hair pins?

- **Bobby pins**—Small pins that create a tight hold on the hair and can be made from plastic or metal that will hold the hair in place. These pins also come in an array of colors, sizes, and decorated designs. In England, bobby pins are also known as hair grips.[7]
- **Hair pins**—Hair pins are similar to bobby pins with more of an open mouth for a looser hold on the hair.[7]

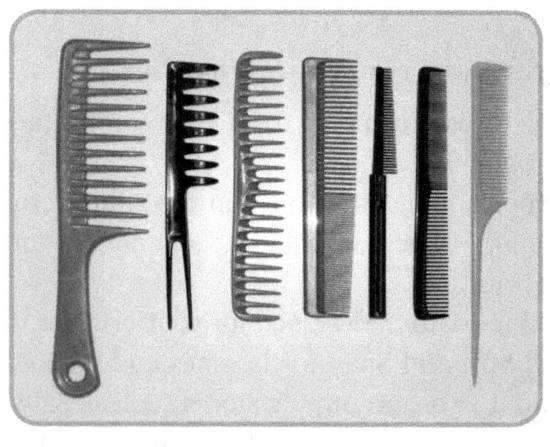

From left to right: wide toothed comb with handle, rake comb, wide toothed comb, large cutting comb, coil comb, small cutting comb, rat tail comb.

What are the best headbands, rubber bands, and pins to use?

This really depends on your hair texture. The best rubber bands I have found are the Ouchless brands because they do not have the metal piece that can snag and tear the hair.

If you have hair that swells and would like to wear headbands you can try the ones that tie in the back or use your own hair to create a braided headband. All other hair textures can usually get away with your average headbands.

Is a water bottle necessary to have?

I believe the water bottle is a great tool. I have two for myself. One bottle has plain water so I can reactivate the products in my hair, and the other has leave-in conditioner. The leave-in conditioner is great after I rinse my hair from a swim or workout and do not have time to shampoo but want to get my hair back into a ponytail or bun.

What are gels?

Gels are normally a jellylike consistency in appearance and feel and create a firm holding style. Many people use gel to slick back the hair or to enhance their natural curl. The drawback to gels is the drying effect it can have on a person's hair.

What are hair mousse/foams?

Hair mousse and foams are very light and resemble whip cream. Mousse is best used on wet hair and can have a firm-to-light holding effect on a hairstyle, depending on the hair texture.

What is hair cream?

Hair cream is just that—cream. It is not a liquid substance that can be sprayed from a bottle but rather scooped out of a container. Creams can be pressing creams, deep conditioners, or hair butters.

What is hair oil?

Oil is a liquid that can be poured from a bottle. Some individuals make their own with different herbs, while others buy their oils, plain or scented, from a store.

What is hair pomade?

Many types of pomade can add shine, slick down, or spike the hair up. It is not a liquid but a solid that can have a smooth or tacky feel.[8]

What is beeswax?

Beeswax is a natural wax secreted by bees to make a honeycomb where bees store their honey. In the hair-care industry, beeswax is usually mixed with other ingredients to hold the hairstyle. Many pomades and hair waxes contain beeswax.

Can I use sunscreen on my natural tress?

I used to apply sunscreen from the health food store in my hair. This was before some companies began to incorporate sunscreen in their products. If you are going to use sunscreen I recommend using organic products because they have a lot less additives that can cause skin irritation.

Chapter 5
WIGS & ADDED HAIR

Though some individuals may feel wigs and added hair do not belong in the natural hair world, they do. Wigs and added hair pieces are a part of various cultures. Some are for religious reasons, stylish reasons, or used to cover the head of a patient who has gone through a traumatic experience. Whatever the reason, it is important to know the basic logistics of these items. In this chapter, I will provide some fundamental definitions and enable the reader to have a better understanding regarding wigs and added hair.

What is a weave/hair extension?

The terms "weave" and "hair extensions" are used interchangeably. Contrary to what many may believe, weaves are not worn only by African American women. Women of all races use weaves/hair extensions. They are strands of human or synthetic hair that can be sewn into the hair or bonded with glue. Extensions can be added to braids, locks, or loose hair for fullness, length, or both.

Can anyone wear weaves/extensions?

No, some individuals, like myself, can be allergic to the hair, while others may have damaged, thin, or fine hair that can be easily irritated or break.

What is the best type of hair to buy when wearing weaves?

Cost usually dictates what people are willing to spend. For instance, human hair can cost more than synthetic, but some individuals prefer human hair because they believe it is not as stripping to their natural hair as synthetic and it is easier to take care of. Synthetic hair is made from man-made fibers, which are intended to look like human hair but do not always achieve that goal. Many synthetic weaves are very shiny and do not blend in well with a person's natural hair. Although new technology is creating better looking and feeling synthetic weaves, they still have a way to go.

Are hair extensions washable?

Human hair extensions have a better chance of holding their form when shampooing than synthetic hair. Many people have complained that synthetic hair tangles and mats when wet, which shortens the wearablity of a hairstyle. If you choose to shampoo your extensions and weaves, read the care label of the hair you bought and the hair products you purchased.

Can I shampoo my wig?

Yes, but it takes practice. I would suggest beginning on an inexpensive wig and reading the instructions of each wig you style because some wigs do not do well without profes-sional styling aids. This will give you the practice you need to become better at wig styling, and at the same time, help you not fear an accident on a wig that is expensive.

Can wigs be styled?

Many wigs can be styled with rollers, curling irons, or pin curls, to name a few. But always read the directions and know what the wig is made from because some wigs can not utilize certain styling aids and products.

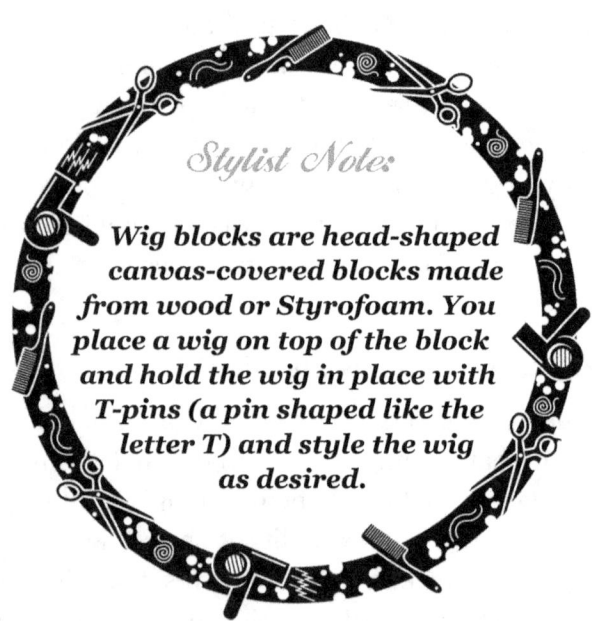

Stylist Note:

Wig blocks are head-shaped canvas-covered blocks made from wood or Styrofoam. You place a wig on top of the block and hold the wig in place with T-pins (a pin shaped like the letter T) and style the wig as desired.

Are weaves damaging?

Weaves can be damaging if sewn or glued in the hair incor-rectly. Here are some ways damaged hair can occur:

- If weaves are sewn in too tightly, the natural hair will pull from the follicle and permanent hair loss from the root can result.
- If an excessive amount of adhesive is used, hair loss can occur during weave removal.
- The thread from the sew-in can put too much tension on the hair and cause the natural hair to snap or weaken.
- If sew-in weaves are used on a constant basis without giving the hair a rest in-between weaves, hair can weaken from the hair follicles.

What does "bonding the hair" mean?

Bonding hair is the same as gluing. The different techniques are:

Stylist Note:

If hair looks weak and sparse after wearing weaves, stop wearing them and seek out a doctor's advice.

- Placing glue on a weft/track and laying the track close to the scalp on a section of hair.
- Using a preglued strand and an instrument that resembles pliers which heats up the glue to melt on your natural hair. This technique is more costly and time-consuming.
- A preglued strip of hair, where the glue is on a piece of tape. When the safety strip is pulled away, it activates the glue to be placed on the hair near the scalp.

What is a wig?

Wigs have been around for thousands of years. They are made of human hair, synthetic, or a combination of both. Some are handmade while others are pieced together by machine. Wigs are one piece and come in an array of colors, styles, and prices.

What is a quick weave?

A quick weave is quick-to-do, hence, the name quick weave. The natural hair is slicked down with gel or braided into cornrows. Next, human or synthetic hair is glued with hair glue (bonding glue/bond adhesive) to the natural mane to create a style. To remove the quick weave, a glue remover (bond remover) is needed to dissolve the bonding adhesive. Many women opt out of this hair technique due to the gel, glue, and removal process which can be sticky and messy because the bonding adhesive can be difficult to completely remove from the hair.

What is a lace-front wig?

Lace fronts are full wigs that have a flap in the front that you can temporarily glue to the skin to blend in with the hairline. Many celebrities prefer lace fronts because if the wig is done properly, it can look flawless.

Are wigs healthy?

Wigs can be a fun way to change your look for a day, week, or month without damaging your natural hair. If you would like to wear wigs I have the following suggestions:

- Do not purchase a cheap wig unless you are wearing it for a costume party.
- Follow the manufacturer's directions on how to wear and take care of the wig.
- Remove the wig when you are home or sleeping to let your scalp breathe.
- Have your wig professionally cleaned if you plan to wear it weekly.
- Treat your real hair with love and care by inspecting your hairline on a weekly basis to avoid hair loss (alopecia).

Do stores sell natural style wigs?

With the rise of women wearing their natural hair, natural style wigs are becoming more popular. I have seen them in specialty stores, hair stores, and online. They range from curly layers to Afros and locks. The possibilities are endless.

Can my natural hair thrive under my wigs and extensions?

With the proper hair care, hair growth should not be an issue. Be sure to shampoo and condition with the appropriate products and always maintain regular trims with your natural tresses. It is also best to have a professional that specializes in weaves address your needs. Not every stylist is skilled enough to install a weave, maintain the natural mane underneath, and communicate with the client about home maintenance. If you feel wearing wigs and extensions is the option for you, be sure to give your hair a rest from artificial hair as often as you can.

What are hair closure pieces?

Hair closures are usually circular or oblong pieces of soft silicone, silk, or lace, and come in many sizes, colors, and hair lengths that have hair attached to them. They are used as a finishing technique to close the top of a sew-in weave. Many closures can be reused if installed properly. They are breathable and very popular with avid weave wearers.

How are closure pieces attached?

Closure pieces are normally attached by sewing the closure piece to a person's hair that was braided down. Some closure pieces have small tiny holes that surround the outskirts of the closure so a needle and thread can easily be pulled through.

Are hair extensions, weaves, and wigs a short-term trend?

Hair extensions, weaves, and wigs have been around since the dawn of time. Wigs have been found in many Egyptian tombs for ceremonial purposes to everyday use. In today's society, movie stars and singers change their looks with hairpieces so they do not damage their own hair, while cancer patients use hairpieces to protect their head from the environment. With this long-standing history of artificial hair use, I do not see weaves or wigs being a passing trend. I believe they are here to stay and will change as technology grows.

What is the difference between hand-tied wefts and machine wefts?

Hand-tied wefts are tied by hand. The hair is knotted by hand onto the *weft* (a long piece of string that looks like it was crocheted with an extremely thin string.) Hand-tied are normally thinner, breathable, and more expensive, which make them more desirable. Machine wefts are sewn with the aid of a machine. The hair is placed onto the weft, and the machine secures the hair to the weft. This can make the weft bulky and noticeable when sewn into the hair. This is why many individuals prefer the hand-tied method to the machine method.

Can hair wefts be split if they have a lot of bulk to them?

Some hair wefts can be split, but splitting the wefts can leave the hairpiece looking sparse. Many individuals will take a scissor or razor and split the weft down the middle. The drawback to splitting the track can be costly because some wefts were designed to be full.

Why do many weave wearers prefer Indian hair to other hair types?

Indian hair is desirable because of its strength, thickness, pliability, and dark color. With these attributes, the hair is easier to style and will last longer with the proper upkeep.

What are Senegalese twists?

Senegalese twists are similar to two-strand twists. The

difference is human or synthetic hair is added to make it fuller and longer.

What are city twists?

City twists are a layered style that resembles two-strand twists and are designed with natural hair extensions, which make them extremely light.

What are tree braids?

Tree braids are designed by adding hair to your natural hair, and as you braid you will leave a few strands of hair out as you go along. This gives the braids a fuller look.

What are block braids?

Block braids are designed with your natural or synthetic hair in a bricklayer pattern. If synthetic hair is used, rollers are usually placed on the ends of the hair, dipped in hot water, and allowed to dry for a clean, finished look.

Chapter 6

CHEMICALS AND THE NATURAL HAIR

Understanding what chemical(s) you are transitioning from can help you better recognize what challenges your hair may have because all chemicals are not created equal. I will touch upon terminology and help you comprehend some basic differences.

What is haircoloring (one word)?

Haircoloring is the act of coloring the hair lighter or darker. Haircoloring is done with permanent, semipermanent, demipermanent chemicals, hair rinses, and hennas.

What is hair color (two words)?

Hair color is a person's natural color.

Who are haircolorists (one word)?

A haircolorist is a person that specializes in coloring hair.

What is a permanent hair color?

Permanent color is considered a chemical color that will not shampoo out of the hair. It can be purchased over-the-counter, or a stylist can apply the color professionally.[1]

What is a semipermanent hair color?

Semipermanent hair color was created to last through several shampoos, depending on hair porosity. It is also known as demipermanent by some manufacturers and is used to deposit color into the hair. Semipermanents are great for women who may want to cover gray and not change the natural color of their nongray hair.[2]

What are highlights and lowlights?

Highlights are achieved when a lighter color is placed in strategic areas of the hair. This gives the effect of lighter hair against darker hair and adds the illusion of sheen and depth. Highlights are normally one to three shades lighter than the darker color in the hair.[3]

Lowlights are the opposite of highlights. Instead of the color being light, the color is dark.

What is color blocking?

Taking a square section or block of hair and applying color can create movement, depth, and shine. A blocking patch can be placed anywhere on the head to make a fashion statement.

What is a hair rinse?

It is a temporary color that is only good from shampoo to shampoo.

What is a color patch test?

This is performed to ensure there are no reactions to any chemicals being used. Some patch tests are administered behind the ear or on the inner part of the elbow.

Can coloring natural hair be damaging?

There are many ways to color natural hair. You can have your hair professionally colored by a licensed cosmetologist, purchase henna, which is plant-based and can be bought over-the-counter, or buy box color that may be plant-based or synthetic and be purchased over-the-counter as well. But in the end, all three can be dangerous if used incorrectly. I find going to a salon with a highly trained stylist that specializes in color is the safest way to have your hair colored. Plus, as a stylist myself, I find when individuals color their hair at home, they tend to miss sections of hair, leaving patches uncolored.

What is henna?

Hennas are natural or vegetable hair colors that are obtained from leaves or the bark of plants. Hennas do not lift the natural hair color and tend to give weak color results. The process can be lengthy and messy, and for this reason, many stylists do not use hennas. The shades range from earth tones, such as, chestnut, and auburn. The major drawback to using hennas can be hair color change. If you choose to change your hair color or want to use a chemical, the results can be inconsistent because the henna coats the hair and does not penetrate the cortex, which can block the chemical process.[4]

Are hennas a good way to condition the hair?

No, hennas only coat the hair cuticle, and traditional hair conditioners penetrate into the cuticle. In other words, the hennas could be giving a person a false conditioning reading. Over time, the buildup on the hair can cause the tresses to be lifeless and difficult to style, so use hennas with caution. Constantly check the status of your hair and remember: if you choose to color your hair later down the line without using hennas, the color could be spotty and inconsistent because it will be hard for a penetrating color to break through the henna dye.

How can I transition out of my hair color?

The color technique used to color the hair can determine the amount of time it will take for the hair to transition and how it will look while transitioning. Transitioning color is not like transitioning out of a relaxer. It differs because the hair texture stays the same when growing out your color. What differs is the color change the hair will go through. The only thing that is similar is how long it may take for color to grow out. Healthy hair can grow one-fourth of an inch to one-half of an inch a month, and depending on the health of the person, your tresses may grow slower or faster.

Here are two scenarios that will help you understand color transitioning:

- Highlights and lowlights may look cleaner to grow out because the whole head is not colored. The high/lowlights are placed strategically to give the hair some depth and movement, and because there are so few it is a cleaner process.
- If the whole head was colored it may be difficult depending on the color. For example, if the hair was colored one to two shades lighter or darker, that means the color is close to your natural color. Your growing-out process will not be too challenging. On the other hand, if you choose a color that was very different from your natural color, you may be in for a long transition.

Why do some stylists like to wait until a person is 100 percent transitioned before coloring their hair?

When an individual has hair that is partially relaxed and partially natural, the color can appear differently on each section and make the hair look damaged and not color uniformly.

Can women color their hair when pregnant?

Yes they can, **but _many women opt out_** of coloring because color is a chemical and due to hormones fluctuating, color can be inconsistent, scalp irritation can occur, and/or excessively dry hair can take place. It is also recommended women stay away from chemicals during pregnancy because COLOR IS A CHEMICAL.

What will swimming do to my hair color?

Depending on the type of water you swim in, your hair color can have a range of issues. The color can fade, especially reds; blonds can become green; hair can become brittle; and split ends can occur. The proper hair-care regimen for your hair texture can help minimize hair fading and split ends. Looking for shampoos and conditioners that say "hydrating" or "for color treated" hair may help as well. If you swim in a pool, look for shampoos that are for pool hair, also known as swimmers' shampoo. These shampoos may help release the chemicals that can become trapped in the hair.

What does a relaxer do to the hair strands?

Relaxers (including children relaxers) break down bonds called disulfide. These bonds make up about one-third of the hair's strength. When the disulfide bonds are broken, the shape is changed permanently and leaves the hair in a weakened state.

Is a permanent wave/cold wave easier on the hair?

No. Disulfide bonds give the hair strength and shape, and these bonds are broken during a permanent wave just as they are during a relaxer. This is how the hair achieves a straight or curly look.

What is a carcinogen?

It is a harmful outside substance that is able to affect the health and well-being of humans and animals. Carcinogens can be found in foods we consume or substances we place on our bodies.[5]

Chapter 7

TRANSITIONING AWAY FROM CHEMICALS

Transitioning away from chemicals can be a daunting task, and without the proper knowledge, many mistakes can easily be made. These questions and answers should head you in the right direction and give you a better understanding on how to transition away from the chemical(s) you have in your hair. Transitioning is a process, and working toward a goal can have its ups and downs, but in the end, the rewards can be glorious.

Do I have to Big Chop (BC), or can I transition?

Believe it or not, you do not have to big chop. Your best defense is a great hair regimen. The first thing you want to do is use organic and natural products to help eliminate the sulfates, propylene glycols, artificial colors, mineral oils, petroleum, and parabens, to name only a few. Without these ingredients, your natural hair will more than likely feel softer and you will not have to fight the tangles and knots that can occur _where your natural hair and relaxer meet, also known as the_ **line of demarcation.**

What is the grow-out method, which is also known as transitioning?

When an individual allows their hair to grow out of their chemically treated hair instead of cutting it off, it is considered transitioning. A person can also transition out of color chemicals too. Individuals who transition will normally have more nonrelaxed hair than chemically treated hair when it is time to cut/trim. This is how transitioning differs from big chopping (BCing).

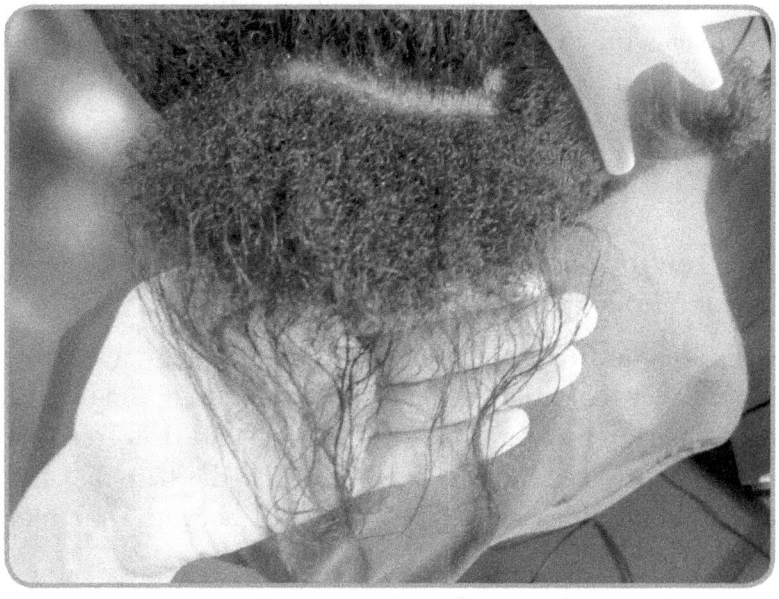

Hair that is transitioning from a relaxer will have straight hair on the ends, and curly hair at the root. Every person will have a different experience transitioning, due to their hair texture and their knowledge of hair.

Are styling options limited when transitioning?

This depends on the texture, length, and health of the hair. Some individuals will have a hard time because their mane is unhealthy and will not hold a style, while others will find transitioning to be a demanding but a doable task.

What is fools' hair?

When an individual decides to **Big Chop (BC)**—_cutting off the chemical that can alter the original hair pattern to expose only the natural hair,_ the first inch and a half may not be your true hair texture. The length of time you have used chemicals on your hair may dictate the length of time you will see your true hair texture and pattern. Some individuals may take up to two years before they can view their natural tresses.

Is a texturizer a good way to transition to natural hair?

This is a question I hear a lot. The answer is no. A texturizer is a relaxer that is left on for a shorter period of time so the hair does not become bone-straight. If a texturizer (relaxer) is constantly used and it overlaps, then the hair that has been chemically treated previously will become straighter over time.

How long does it take to completely transition to natural?

Healthy natural hair can grow one-fourth to one-half of an inch a month. If you have short hair, it will take you no time at all to transition, but the longer the hair the more time you will need if you are not willing to stay on track with your hair trims.

A great example I use for my clients over the years is this:

If you have three inches of chemically treated hair, then it can take you up to six months or more to be natural. But if you have six inches of chemically treated hair, it may take you up to one year or more to grow out the chemical. The longer the hair, the longer the transition time.

Does hair pattern play a part in the ease of transitioning?

Yes, I believe it does if you are not used to handling natural hair. As a licensed cosmetologist, I have seen many different hair textures, even on the same person's head. I have noticed when women have supertight curls, it can be a little challenging to keep the natural curly hair from not tangling with the relaxer when shampooing.

If hair is extremely damaged from chemicals and the individual does not want to cut the hair, the chemically treated hair will tangle and become difficult to comb through, especially if the natural hair is tight. However, if the natural hair has more of a wave, it may be easier to transition because the hair is not curling over itself. If you have very tight curls, be sure to use extra conditioner. I like water-based leave-in conditioning sprays after your normal shampoo and conditioning routine. This should help with breakage and tangling.

Why does my hair seem to be breaking now that I have transitioned?

As you transition, you will realize chemically treated hair is just that, chemically treated. When hair is wet, it can stretch up to 50 percent. If hair has lost its elasticity due to dryness or from being chemically treated, breakage can occur. Natural hair, on the other hand, is the healthy hair and very rarely will you see natural hair break unless it is undergoing trauma such as dryness.

A great point to remember: The curlier the hair, the more likely you will have breakage. Curly hair has bends and curves to it, which can trap the natural **sebum** *(hair oils)* in the pockets of hair. This will not allow the sebum to reach the ends, causing drying and breakage.[1]

How can I tell if I am losing my natural hair or my relaxed hair is breaking while I am transitioning?

Normally, if you are losing hair, you will see the scalp and the hair will not occupy the hair follicle. In this case, be sure to consult your doctor. *A STYLIST CANNOT HELP YOU!*

If the relaxed hair is breaking, you will have hair in the follicle but will see where the relaxer has separated (broken) from the natural hair. Normally the hair will break at the **line of demarcation**—*where the natural hair and chemical meet.*

When is the best time to cut the chemicals from the hair?

I believe this answer will vary for many different reasons because there are many different hair textures. Therefore, I will answer this question in more than one way.

a. When the new growth and the relaxer begin to tangle after shampooing this is an indication the two textures are not going to get along. The tighter the curl pattern, the sooner you may have to cut the chemical from the hair because the two textures are so different it makes styling difficult.

b. If the hair has a natural wave, not a tight curl, it may be easier to grow out the relaxer because the two textures are not that far apart.

c. If you are trying to grow out your relaxer but blow-dry your hair on extreme heat, it can alter the new growth. This makes it hard to distinguish the new growth from the chemically treated hair. At this point, you may want to cut the relaxer off to protect the integrity of the natural hair.

d. When you feel comfortable with the length that has grown in. Some people do not mind short hair, but others may want the minimum of three inches so they can have some shape and style to their hair.

e. It's time if you begin to see a lot of hair breakage on the floor or your clothing.

Is roller setting the hair a good way to transition?

This depends on the length, health, and texture of hair, but overall, I say yes, because wet sets put less stress on the hair and the *line of demarcation—(where the chemical and natural hair meet).* You may also change your look with different-size curls which can be achieved with various sized rollers.

Can I transition out of my chemically treated hair with weaves, wigs, and braids?

Transitioning with weaves, wigs, and braids can be tricky, and this is why I do not recommend it. I have observed many women transitioning with artificial hair only to be frustrated in the end. The false hair does not allow the individual to understand the way their hair grows from the scalp, and when it is removed, it is difficult to fall into a hair regimen because they may not understand how their curls grow in the beginning. This can result in a person going back to a relaxer.

Chapter 8

SHAMPOOING, CONDITIONING & HAIR TREATMENTS FOR TRANSITIONERS

Transitioning away from chemicals can be stressful, but when you add shampooing your own hair into the mix, it can be frightening. I find understanding the basic knowledge about cleaning and conditioning transitioning hair can ease the pain of home maintenance and make your transitioning stage bearable.

What is the best way to shampoo hair that is in the transitioning state?

Shampooing with a moisturizing or hydrating shampoo will help cut back tangles in the hair. Detangling with a conditioner before you wet the hair can cut the tangle process because some hair textures become more knotted when wet. If your hair is long, you can section the hair in two and shampoo. It will help you not become overwhelmed.

You can part your hair from ear to ear, or from the forehead to the nape of the neck in a straight line. If you section from ear to ear, be sure to shampoo the top half first. By shampooing the top section of your head first, it ensures the soap will not run back into the section that was previously cleaned.

Will I have to use two separate shampoos?

Let me start by saying, it depends on the hair texture and what you are willing to put up with. If you have a tight curl pattern, you may have to use two shampoos when the hair begins to grow longer. If you have a dry scalp or dandruff, it will be best to shampoo with the dandruff shampoo first because it can sometimes make the hair tangle. By using the hydration shampoo second, it can help reduce the knots before the conditioner is used.

Should I comb my hair before shampooing?

If at all possible, yes, this will help the hair not to tangle or knot up when it becomes wet. Using a wide-toothed comb or a pick are the best tools to use when combing the hair. Some individuals will apply conditioner to the hair before they begin to detangle. Conditioner helps the comb glide through the hair much easier.

Are deep conditioners good for transitioning hair?

Yes, the proper conditioner can never hurt any hair texture. Conditioners are used to add moisture back into the hair. If the hair feels dry and/or brittle, by all means condition away. Deep conditioners can also lessen hair breakage when transitioning.

What are the benefits of hair steamers?

Hair steamers were designed to add moisture to the hair by using heat and steam vapors to open the cuticles of hair while conditioning molecules penetrate. Some haircolorists use steamers to add colors into the hair. Though some individuals like hair steamers, others do not. Some people have had bad experiences and claim steamers loosen the hair from the follicle and cause more hair shedding than normal, leaving the hair looking and feeling sparse. From a professional standpoint, I do understand this because when you steam your face, it allows your pores to expand so you can extract blackheads. The same thing may be said with hair follicles. If you steam the hair, does that allow the hair to loosen from the follicle and be extracted when brushing? At this point in time, testing has not been done on this theory. For many individuals, the verdict on hair steamers is still out for debate. If you feel you need to have the conditioner penetrate the hair, try a heating cap or a plastic cap with a towel wrapped around the plastic cap. It will hold in your body temperature (which the body regulates naturally) and allows the conditioner to penetrate into the hair without artificial heat. You can also sit in a hot steamy bathroom which can do the same thing for a fraction of what a hair steamer may cost.

Chapter 9

GENERAL INFORMATION
FOR LOCKED HAIR

Taking care of locked hair does not have to be difficult. In this section, I will give general information to key questions many of my clients had over the years that pertain to swimming with locks to the uniqueness of them. You will find many of the answers straightforward and a wealth of knowledge for your personal peace of mind.

What should I know before I lock my hair?

Know that you have options to many different nonlocked styles, and if you want to lock your hair, you can with different techniques. When individuals approach me for a consultation or stop me at a function, I encourage them to wear their hair nonlocked first. I want the individual to experience all aspects of being natural. Wearing their natural tresses will help them make a sound decision without regrets in the future. I do feel some individuals rush into locks because they do not understanding the beauty of their natural texture and feel locks are the only option. I also like to stress that locks are low maintenance, but still need care. I see many individuals make the mistake of locking because they feel they do not have to shampoo or care for the hair, which is false. Hair, regardless of the texture, must be cared for to see optimal results.

Who are loctitians?

Loctitians are individuals who maintain and groom locks. Some loctitans will also style, color, and cut the locks into a design.

What are the different techniques to locking hair?

Traditional/ single twist: The hair can be twisted with a comb, palm rolled, or finger twisted. When the hair sheds, it will shed into the lock. Traditional locks form by the hair coiling around itself, and over time, intertwines with the same hair it has coiled around.

Stylist Note:

Some states do not have laws on natural hairstyling, so if you are looking for someone that is licensed, please keep in mind if you do not ask the right questions and your hair is destroyed, you may not have a case in court.

There are **three** stages of traditional lock formation.

1. **Twist:** The hair is not locked but is twisted with a comb or fingers that forms a coil and can be

shampooed loose. Twists can also frizz and sweat out if hot outside or if a person perspires heavily.[1]

2. **_Teenage/Budding Stage:_** This is the stage where many people who are locking feel the most frustration. The hair begins to form little buds that feel like a soft spongy eraser. Teenage/Budding Stage is the first stage of locking. At this point, some hair textures can be combed out, but I would not recommend doing this. You do not want the hair to undergo stress from combing. This may cause you to restart the locking process from the twist stage again.[2]

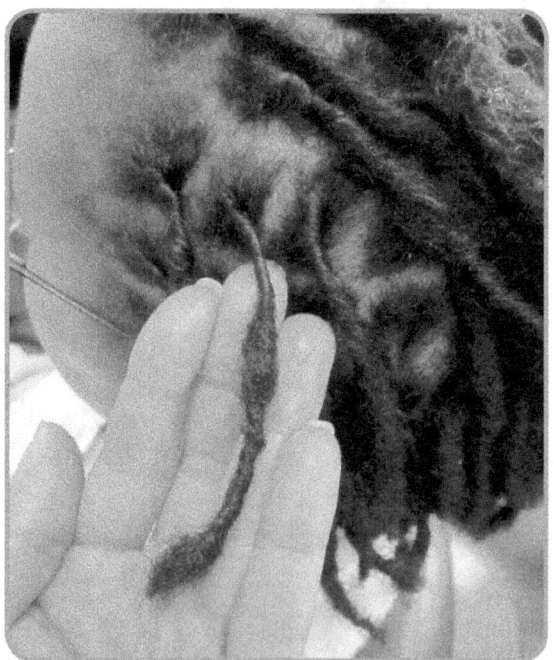

Hair was hand twisted to create these locks. Over time, the hair began to intertwine with itself and a spongy lump appeared. This is also known as budding.

3. **Mature Locks:** The locks have intertwined over time and cannot be combed out without hair loss. At this stage, you can shampoo without the hair unraveling at the ends and styling will be easier and more frequent.[3]

Two-strand twist: Two pieces of hair are twisted around each other to make the hair resemble a rope braid. As the new hair grows at the root, it can be twisted by palm rolling or finger twisting. It would be best to twist all the way down to ensure the ends of the hair will not open or unravel.

Braiding: The hair is braided and as it grows it is retwisted (maintained) the same as the two-strand twist would be.[3]

Extension lock: There are many ways to install extension locks, but it is the same premise as the two-strand twist and braiding technique. When I did extension locks, I would just shampoo, retwist, clip, and set under the dryer to dry.

Interlocking/latching/Sisterlocks[TM]**:** These techniques are similar in the way they are maintained. With a hook and an interweaving method a lock can be formed.

Latching, interlocking, or Sisterlocks®: The hair is intertwined within itself with a tool such as a crochet hook to form links. Sisterlocks® are a registered trademark company.

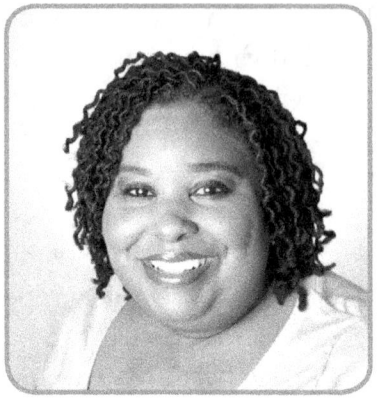

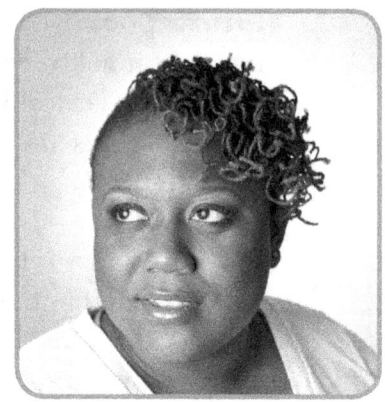

Here are beautiful palm rolled locks that were set on rods, and over time the curls dropped to give the locks a crimped looked.

Locks come in many different shapes and sizes. Our model, Nakisha, wears her sisterlocks full in the bang area

How can I choose the best locking technique for my hair?

Here is a rule of thumb I have used for years with my clients.

- *Straight Hair*—Ratting the hair with a comb, and then using a crochet hook to interlock or knot the hair.
- *Wavy Hair*—Depending on the depth of the wave, you could use the same technique as straight hair, extensions, braids, or coils.
- *Curly Hair*—You can twist/coil the hair, interlock, braid, two-strand twist, or use extensions.
- *Tightly Coiled*—You can twist/coil the hair, interlock, braid, two-strand twist, or use extensions.

What is the best size for a lock?

Hair density (the amount of hair in an area) and the strength of the hair determine the size of the lock. Some individuals will go with the size they feel is best for their styling needs, which is fine, but remember, if your roots cannot support the weight of the lock, you may want to stay away from locks that are too small or too big.

What makes locks unique for each person?

Hair texture, density, locking technique, and maintenance techniques are the reasons locks can look different from person to person.

What is lock separation?

After shampooing the hair, exercising, or just grooming, the locks should be separated from one another so they do not stick together. For the person that likes to have their hair parts showing all the time, this is especially important. Lock separation is also vital for the person that may have a sensitive scalp, also known as being tender-headed. If the locked hair has not been separated during the shampoo process, it can pull on the scalp when it is time to groom the hair and cause the locks to become weak.[4]

What is splitting the locks?

Splitting the lock is cutting the lock in half from the ends to the roots. It can be a difficult task depending on the length and age of the lock. The longer the lock the harder it can be to split the lock because the lock has been intertwined longer and is harder to separate. Older locks can be cut down the middle, which would leave a straight line, resulting in the locks taking on a half moon appearance. This technique can cause the locks to unravel because it has disturbed the hair's intertwinement. If possible, refrain from splitting locks if the locks are mature.

Can I pick lint out of my locks?

When lint intertwines with locks it becomes part of the hair, and if picked out, it can weaken the locked hair. Lint should only be taken off the hair if it is lying on top of the lock so it will not unravel or weaken the lock. Some people feel the white lint in their hair is unsightly so they choose to color their hair to minimize the lint. Depending on the texture and the coloring technique used, you will not be able to tell lint was trapped in the locks.

Will doubling locks be harmful to my hair?

Some individuals double their locks because the locks were made too small or they have lost a lock or two and do not want an empty space in their hair. Whatever the reason, be sure that doubling is what you want to do because it is a lot easier combining than splitting locks. From my professional standpoint, I try to steer my clients away from doubling unless the lock cannot withhold the weight of the base it is on. When the lock is double be sure to cut the weakest one off. This will ensure the base to the one you just doubled stands firm.[5]

Can I pick out my locks and keep the length of my hair?

No, locks are hair that has been twisted or interlocked. When natural shedding occurs, it will shed into the lock and help the locking process. If you try to pick them out, you may find your hair will be on the floor and shorter than you have anticipated.

Why do locks turn a lighter color?

Locked hair is a style that has been either intertwined or interlocked with hair. When locked hair is styled with either of these two methods, it does not have the chance to shed from the hair. It actually becomes part of the lock; therefore, the hair is dead and is predisposed to color change.

Why are my locks beginning to thin out?

Some people notice their locks thinning over time and cannot comprehend why. While I am not a doctor and cannot determine a medical reason, I can give you some guidance. Here are a few suggestions to consider:

- The hair is being retightened too tight, and it is being pulled from the follicle.
- A person may have started a new medication that affects their hair.
- As you age, hair texture may change and naturally thin.
- The locks have grown very long and the root (or anchor) cannot hold the weight of that lock.
- Excessive styling that pulls the roots, such as buns or

ponytails that are too tight, can thin locks.
- Harsh chemicals such as color can also be the culprits.
- Your locks aged. Yes, locks age, like people, and separate from a section of the lock.

Why do some locks detach or fall out?

There are many reasons for a lock to detach from the head.

Here are some reasons:

- Over twisting at the root can cause weakening of the root.
- Pulling the locks taut when styling. This can cause weak point either at the root or anywhere throughout the lock.
- Not maintaining the hair properly can cause the locks to have weak points.
- Trimming up the lock too early during the locking process will not allow the hair to wrap around the lock and cause it to take longer to lock and intertwine.
- They were made too small when started and over time the weight was too much for the root/base to hold.
- Locks were shaved or trimmed up the shaft too early which caused weak points through the locks because the hair did not have time to wrap itself around the forming lock.

Can I cut my locks into a style?

Of course, as long as they are mature! I have had the pleasure of cutting layers, creating cute bobs, and even shaving one side. You are limited only to your imagination.

Can I transition out of my locks to an Afro?

Yes, I have transitioned many of my clients out of their locks. I like to grow the hair out about two to three inches, and that means not retightening the root. The texture will determine the amount of hair a person may want to grow out. I suggest two to three inches to have some hair to play with, and, before you know it, you will have enough new growth for a rod set, coil-out, or both, depending on the hair texture.

Can I sleep on wet locks?

No. Locks are a cylinder shape that can flatten out over time if they are slept on wet. Plus, depending on the thickness of the locks, if not dried properly, they can begin to have a mildew odor.

What are the drawbacks to having locks?

- Mildew odor if not dried properly.
- If too long, you can sit on them and your neck will jerk back.
- If pulled or styled too tight, traction alopecia can occur.
- If not maintained properly, weak points can occur throughout the locks.

Will I have freedom with locks?

Freedom is a state of mind. I have many friends with locks, and they feel great. Overall, they say they save money by not going to the hair salon as often. Their hair seems healthier without the constant combing, and it is low maintenance; plus, styling options are plenty.

Can a person with locked hair go swimming?

In short, yes. If locked hair is matured, I would suggest braiding the hair back in a cornrow style or in individual plaits. This is an easy way for the hair not to be disrupted too much and cut back on the frizz. No matter how the hair was worn while swimming, it is very important to rinse the hair with fresh water so chemicals or salt do not disrupt the intertwinement of the locks. It is also very important to dry the locked hair so a mildew odor does not set in.

Should children wear locks?

This depends on the culture the individual is from. I would not say no to someone if locks are a part of their custom, but I may tell a parent to consider the long-term outcome. I would also remind the parent that locks would have to be cut off in order to be removed. This may not be a big deal if you have a boy, but if you have a girl and her hair has grown long, it could be a shock when it is time to cut them off. You may also want to consider the overall cost and time you and the child will have to put in.

What is a forked lock?

It is a lock that has two tails and one point of origin at the base. Forked locks normally happen when two locks are combined/married together. If you do not like the look of forked locks you can cut off the weakest end.[6]

What is the controversy with using the word dreadlock?

The region you live in can determine the positive or negative connotation of this word. Many individuals that I run into do not like the word *dreadlocks* because they feel there is nothing *dreadful* about their locks, while others do not mind the word *dreadlock*. Because I style hair for a living I like to play it safe, so I use the word *locks* or *locs*. Either spelling is acceptable.

Chapter 10

SHAMPOOING, CONDITIONING & TREATMENTS FOR LOCK

Clean hair is essential to healthy hair, and it is no different with locked hair. No matter what stage of locking the hair, it must be shampooed and conditioned. This will ensure you have healthy locks and product buildup will not occur.

Is it possible to shampoo during the locking process?

In short, yes. Shampooing is part of the locking process, especially with traditional locks. Shampooing may not be a weekly event with traditional locks, but it is a must. Clean hair is important for health reasons. Hair can attract dirt and buildup that carry germs and must be cleansed of them. This is why I recommend shampooing biweekly. Look for clarifying shampoos or shampoos that are made with natural organic botanicals that are not creams. Creams can be difficult to shampoo out of the hair and can cause hair to slip, which you are trying to avoid. What many individuals do not know is that by shampooing every two weeks you are training the hair to stay in its parts and thus, create a lock. *You do not need to avoid shampooing for this process to take place.*[1]

How often should my locks be shampooed?

When you shampoo traditional locks they will unravel at the root and will need to be retwisted. Many of my clients with traditional locks shampoo every two to three weeks because shampooing every day is not feasible. On the other hand, if you have locks that are latched/interlocked, you can shampoo more often without worrying the roots will unravel. My clients with interlocking locks normally will shampoo once or twice a week because of scalp issues or because they work out.

What is the best way to shampoo and condition locked hair?

Shampooing locks are a lot easier than one may believe. Many of my clients who need to shampoo their hair at home simply do this with four items: A water bottle, noncream shampoo, an applicator bottle, and leave-in conditioning spray.

Try not to use shampoos that have a heavy cream base. These shampoos will be hard and sometimes impossible to completely rinse out of the hair. You want to use shampoos that are water-based and/or clear. I strongly suggest putting your shampoo in a bottle that has an applicator tip on it. This way, you can place the shampoo where you would like with just a gentle squeeze. When you are done, take a water bottle filled with warm water and spray in between your parts where you have placed the shampoo. Last, with your fingertips, massage for a minimum of five minutes. Rinse and repeat as often as you need to. As far as conditioners go, I suggest organic water-based spray leave-in conditioners. I find they do not leave a buildup and soften the hair just as well as cream-based products.

What is spot cleaning?

Spot cleaning is another way to clean sections of your scalp without a complete shampoo. This is normally done with a washcloth and warm water. Some individuals will use shampoo, a water-apple cider vinegar mix, or just water depending on the scalp issues they may have.[2]

Why do some individuals with locks have a mildew odor?

Locks can retain moisture and the odor stems from hair that was not properly dried. The best way to rid the hair from odor is the use of clarifying shampoos, which contain vinegar. Next, dry the hair completely by sitting under a hooded dryer. If the odor is strong, shampoo the hair more frequently. If the odor is very intense, it can take months to correct the problem.[3]

Are hot oil treatments good for locks?

I do not agree with using hot oil on locks. Simply put, the locks can separate and loosen the intertwinement and become puffy. Depending on the texture of hair, the locks can unravel quickly.

Should locks be steamed?

In my professional opinion, I say no. I have seen locks that have been steamed and they unravel over time. Steam swells the hair and can cause the locks to unravel. I have also witnessed weak points throughout some individuals' locks because during their locking process, the hair was not started properly, and due to poor maintenance, left the hair with weak points throughout the locks.

Are hair masks good for locked hair?

No. Locks are hair that have been matted or interlocked together, which means hair sheds into the lock. That being said, if you put a mask on locks, it may be difficult to shampoo out and can cause buildup. If you would like softer locks, try a water-based leave-in conditioner spray, but remember, locks are dead hair that has shed into a long string of hair and there is not much you can do to make them soft.

Are dandruff treatments healthy for locks?

Dandruff treatments do not interfere with locks unless you do not rinse them out properly or a water-based leave-in spray conditioner does not follow the dandruff shampoo. Some medications are very strong and can strip the hair of its moisture. This is the reason for a water-based leave-in conditioning spray.

Can lock extensions be shampooed?

Yes, they can, but before you receive lock extensions, it is best to consult with the stylist who will perform the service and ask if their method is washable. Some extensions are sewn in, braided in, or crocheted, and depending on the experience of the stylist, this can dictate how long the extension will last and if they are washable.

Chapter 11

LOCK STYLING QUESTIONS

Locks can be styled for all occasions, including work, and look great too. Styling options are only limited to your imagination and having fun with them should be included as well. Never feel that you are shortchanged because you have chosen to lock your hair.

Are styling products good for locks?

I find that less is best and nothing is better when it comes to locks. Many individuals believe you have to use products for the hair to lock, but if you revisit the question, *"What are the different techniques to locking hair?"* you will find one of those methods will work best for your hair texture. I prefer not to use products to retwist my client's roots. I would shampoo, use a water-based leave-in conditioning spray, retwist, and use clips to hold the twisted lock into place. After the hair is clipped, you need to sit under the dryer until the hair is 100 percent dried, and then the clips can be removed and the hair is done.

Can locks be styled?

Yes. Locks can be braided, rod set, set in an updo, and

twisted around each other, just to name a few styles. You are truly limited only to your imagination.

Can locks be curled?

Yes, locks can be curled. The size and style you would like dictates the kind of roller that should be used. Many people use perm rods or the wrap-a-loc roller to get a nice tight curl that will last.

What does shaving, cleaning, or up-trimming locks mean?

This refers to when you take some scissors or a clipper, hold the lock in your hand, and cut the wild stray hairs that stick out from the lock. This makes the locks more manageable in styling and helps prevent wild-looking locks. Many people who work in the corporate world prefer to clean their locks because it gives them a finished, professional look.

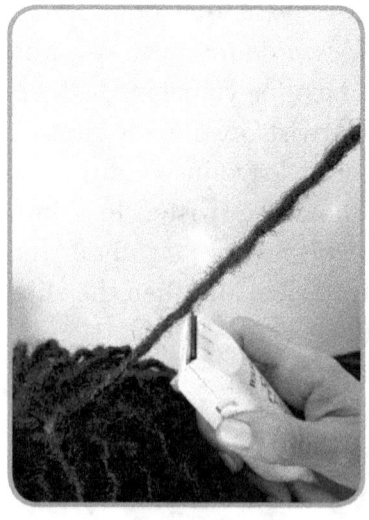

This lock will have its wild hairs clipped from the shaft to give it a smoother and cleaner appearance. Cleaning the shaft will also help locks maintain its style longer.

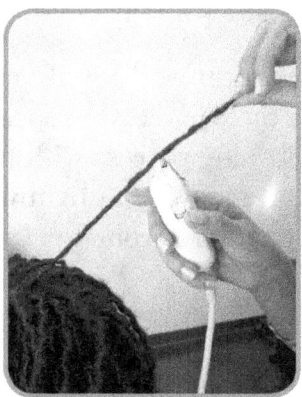 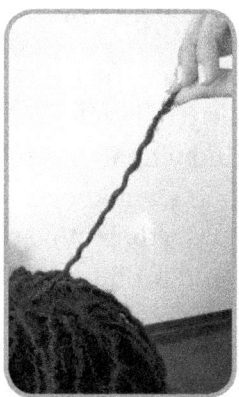

The lock's shaft has been clipped, beginning from the root and ending on the tip.

The lock's shaft is completely clipped, and the remnants of an old rod set can now be seen.

Can you style hair that is in the budding stage?

Yes, depending on the length of hair. Remember, locks can be started in many different ways, and if you have medium-to-long hair, you have some length to play with. In the budding stage of some lock styles, I have seen people cornrow their locks, curl the locks, and simply pin the locks to make curls or buns.

What are geni-locs?

This occurs when yarn is wrapped around a braid to resemble locks. Some people will wrap different color yarn around their locks for a more fashionable and trendy look. Geni-locks are removable. This is great for the person that decides they only want locks for vacation or a special event.

What is nudred?

Nudred is a spongelike hair tool that works well on short, extracurly hair. The tool gives the curls a coil appearance. Some individuals begin their locking process with the nudred tool. I would encourage anyone who has tightly coiled hair to visit their Web site, www.nudred.com, to view their videos and product.

Chapter 12
LOCKS & COLOR

Despite what people think, locks can be colored. Though color is a chemical, it is a choice many women choose to embrace because of fashion reasons or just to cover gray. Whatever the justification, it is important to understand what color can do to your locks and the choices a lock wearer has when contemplating coloring their locks.

Can locks be colored?

Locks can be colored dark or made honey blond depending on the thickness, but it is very different coloring locks than natural hair because locks are dead hair that are intertwined within themselves. When hair is locked, it sheds into the lock, and that can prevent an even hair tone.

If a lock is very thin, you may want to rethink a color that is in the blond family because it requires a strong lifting agent called a developer. Developers come in many different strengths and a stylist can control the lightening process.

Can over-the-counter color be used on locks?

Color is a chemical, and I do not promote individuals using

chemicals. Box color also comes in one formula: strong. A licensed stylist can adjust the strength of the formula and the tone of the color, which you cannot do with a box color.

Does coloring damage locks?

If done _incorrectly_, color can damage any hair type, locks included.

If I color my locks darker, can I lighten them if I choose to go lighter?

Locks are hair that has intertwined/matted over time. This means there will be strands of hair that have shed into the lock and are no longer attached to the scalp. For this reason, once you color your locks dark, it is hard to lift to a lighter color without weakening the locks. One important point to remember is prolonged bleach use can destroy your hair so it is something I highly discourage.

Can I color my gray hair without changing the color of my natural lock color?

Yes, a professional has the tools to cover the gray, but I have not found an over-the-counter product to cover the gray and not change the natural hair color.

Why are the ends of my locks lighter than the middle and shaft of my locks?

The hair that is further away from the scalp is exposed to the environment longer and can tend to lighten from the sun, harsh shampoos, or overuse of products.

Will hair bleach be harsh on my locks?

The size of the locks and the harshness of the lightener determine if you can use hair lightener. I have used bleach on locks before and never had a problem, but remember, as a professional, I have access to mild to high lift lightening products.

Stylist Note:

Be careful of hennas. Hennas are plant-based colors that come in brown, blue, and reddish tones. Hennas coat the hair and do not penetrate, which can cause a film on a person's locks.

If the locks are very thin, I would suggest steering clear from bleaches because the bleach can destroy or weaken the locked hair. If the locks are thick, proceed with caution, but overall, when it comes to chemicals, find an experienced licensed stylist that can give your hair the love and attention it needs to proceed with chemicals.

Can highlights be obtained with hair that is locked?

Yes, highlights are achieved when color is placed in strategic areas of the head. This gives the effect of light hair against dark hair. To accomplish great results, an experienced colorist should be able to reach the color a client desires.

Do hennas work well with locked hair?

I find individuals who used hennas for their locks had a tough time shampooing the henna completely out of the hair. Also, if the lock color should try to be lightened later, the lighter color may not penetrate the henna because hennas coat the hair, which leaves it hard for hair products to penetrate to the cuticle of the hair strand. Also, if bleach is used to remove henna-treated locks, the color may be spotty and inconsistent.

Chapter 13

THE NATURAL HAIR BRIDE

Weddings are a time for great celebrations and having natural hair should not be an issue when getting married. There are more than enough styles to choose from if you open your mind.

How do I choose a hairstyle for my wedding day?

Choosing a style is not as hard as many may think. I have found if you have an ornate dress, then the style should be simple. The dress and the hair should never compete. Both should always complement each other.

The weather is another consideration. Be mindful of the hair texture you possess because if you have curly hair and blow it out straight on a hot humid day, the hair will frizz and could be dreadful in pictures. Also, test hairstyles on yourself. It does not have to be perfect. You just want to get an idea of what you may or may not like for your special day.

Can a bride wear a short haircut?

Many brides feel a style should be elaborate and classic, but the truth is, times have changed and the definition of classic hairstyles along with it. I do not think because you are a bride you have to wear your hair long. That is like telling a man he cannot wear his hair long, locked, or in cornrows for his wedding day. Think outside the box and keep your mind open. The possibilities may surprise you. Many women wear their hair in two-strand twists or a simple coil-out with a hairpiece that sparkled with rhinestones. Short hair is what you make of it, so make it dazzle.

How can I wear my hair under a veil?

A veil can be a great addition to any wedding dress, and when it comes to hairstyle-veil combos, that can become tricky. I suggest thinking about the wedding as a whole. Will you keep the veil on all night, or will you take it off half-way through the night? Answering these questions will help you decide on the style you will choose for your special day. For the most part, the dress will help you decide the style that will be appropriate for you, and veils can be worn on hair that is short, long, up, or down. Veils can be handmade from a piece of jewelry or attached to a crown or pillbox hat. You are only restricted to your imagination. If you choose to wear a veil, practice with different looks seven to ten weeks before the wedding. This will ensure you have had enough time to find the look that suits you on your special day.

Can something else beside a veil be worn?

Yes. Hats, flowers, feathers, and jewelry—whatever you feel will fit your personality and style. Some individuals will chose not to wear a hairpiece and let the hairstyle speak for itself.

What is a formal updo?

A formal updo normally has a clean appearance and the hair is worn up and off the neck. You can see these styles worn at proms, weddings, and other formal events.

What is a semi-updo?

Semi-updos are great for women with long hair. The hair is normally pinned up in the front while the back cascades in curls, braids, waves, or is straight. Semi-updos can be worn anywhere, anytime, and are great to keep your hair off your face. I find any texture can have a semi-updo and look great.

Can locks be lengthened for a bridal hairstyle?

Yes, but go to a specialist that deals with lock extensions. There are many ways to add on to your mane, and choosing the right technique is very important because if it is only for your wedding day, you may want to make sure the extensions do not damage your natural hair when you take them out.

Chapter 14
NATURAL HAIR IN THE WORKPLACE

Over the years many corporations and universities have changed polices on various issues. Hairstyling is one of the subjects that have adjusted with time. Back in the 1980s and early 1990s, many African American women fought to keep their jobs or did not accept certain positions because cultural tolerance was not equal. Some women also felt they did not want to compromise their cultural identity.[1]

As times have changed, so have some of the strict rules on hair grooming and clothing attire. I remember when there was no such thing as wearing jeans to work, but that seems to be the norm in some businesses nowadays. I can also recall my high school years, when braids in a predominantly white school would get you looks of wonder.

Are braids a good style for work?

This depends on the style itself because some braids are designed with your own hair while other styles have hair added. Due to some jobs, extensions may be a danger if working with highly flammable materials. Be sure to look into the work rules and regulations. The same can be said about facial hair with men.

Are Afros acceptable to wear to work?

I love this question for many reasons, and the answer is yes, as long as the Afro has style and shape. Do not think you can walk into a job regardless of the title and have an unkempt mane. Natural or not, your hair should look professional, and that means clean and styled.

Are locks acceptable in corporate America?

Over the years, locks as well as natural hair have been getting the thumbs-up in corporate America. Some companies have rewritten their handbooks to incorporate rules and regulations on grooming. Some of the new regulations suggest a good appearance is a clean one and mention very little or nothing about the kind of hairstyle that is to be worn. On the other side of the coin, you may run into some corporations that will frown upon locked hair. This depends on the CEOs of the company and where and how their views of beauty stand.

Will I get hired with locks?

As long as they are neat I do not see why not. I have clients that are doctors, lawyers, and teachers who sport long beautiful locks. On the other hand, I do think safety issues can arise when certain jobs are involved. A very good friend of mine cut his locks off when he became a firefighter because he felt they would be a safety hazard for him. I am not saying you cannot express your right to wear the hairstyle of your choice; just consider the safety aspect of any style before you invest time and money.

I have coworkers who want to touch my natural hair during work hours. How can I explain to them with tact I do not like my hair touched?

I think the key word is *tact*. After all, you do not want to lose your job over another person's ignorance. I would respectfully suggest they cannot, and let them know your hair is part of your personal space and you feel uncomfortable with that request. Because you are at work, keep it professional. Give them an example of how your hair may feel, e.g., like cotton, wool, or a satin material. It does not matter if you work on Wall Street or for a fast-food company. This will show the individual who asked the question you do not mind inquiries, but it is a request you cannot honor.

References

Chapter 1—100 Percent Natural: General Information

[1] Bonner, Lonnice Brittenum. *Plaited Glory: For Colored Girls Who've Considered Braids, Locks, and Twists.* Three River Press, 31, 1996.

[2] Massey, Lorraine, with Michele Bender. *Curly Girl.* Thomas Allen & Son Limited, 14. 2010.

[6] Massy, 97.

[7] Massy, 14.

[3] Walker, Andre. *Andre Talks Hair!* Simon & Schuster, 45, 1999.

[4] Central Centrifugal Cicatricial Alopecia—Hampton University Skin of Color Research Institute *http://huscri.org/resources/patient-information/ccca/* Last Viewed February 25, 2013.

[5] Hantash, Basil M., M.D., Ph.D., Robert A. Schwartz, M.D., MPH. "Traction Alopecia: Cause and Treatment Options": *http://traction-alopecia.com/* Last Viewed February 25, 2013.

[8] "Satin or Silk Pillowcases for Hair and Face"—Info Barrel Lifestyle *http://www.infobarrel.com/Satin_or_Silk_Pillowcase_for_Hair_and_Face/* Last Viewed February 25, 2013.

[9] "Keratin Hair Treatment: What to Expect"—WebMd *http://www.webmd.com/healthy-beauty/features/keratin-hair-straightening-treatments/* Last viewed February 19, 2013.

[10] "Water and Humans"—Water Facts *http://www.water-info.org/resources/water-facts/* Last Viewed February 20, 2013.

Chapter 2—Shampooing, Conditioning & Hair Treatments for 100 Percent Naturals

[1] Kinard, Tulani. *No Lye!* St. Martin's Press, 43, 1997.

[2] Bailly, Jenny. "The 5 biggest hair myths". *http://www.cnn.com/2012/01/13/living/hair-myths-0/* Last viewed February 25, 2013.

[3] "Soft Water vs. Hard Water for Hair" *http://www.livestrong.com/article/70873-soft-water-vs.-hard-water/* Last viewed on February 25, 2013.

[4] Bonner, Lonnice Brittenum. *Plaited Glory: For Colored Girls Who've Considered Braids, Locks, and Twists.* Three River Press, 33, 1996.

[5] "The Most Popular Natural Preservatives"—*Natural*

Cosmetic News http://www.naturalcosmeticnews.com/ new-ingredients/the-most-popular-natural-preserva- tives-2/ Last Viewed February 25, 2013.

[6] Down, R. (2013). "The Buzz, Natural Rx Kit." (3rd ed., Vol. 39, 22). San Francisco: *Vegetarian Times*/ Last viewed February 26, 2013.

Chapter 3—Styling Questions
[1] Bonner, Lonnice Brittenum. *Plaited Glory: For Colored Girls Who've Considered Braids, Locks, and Twists*. Three River Press, 38, 1996.

[11] Bonner, 76 & 86.

[12] Bonner, 76.

[13] Bonner, 78.

[2] Parson, Martin. Martin Parson's Long Hair Secrets, Volume 1. Intermar Productions, 20, 2006.

[3] Rennells, Lauren. *Vintage Hairstyling Retro Styles with Step-by-Step Techniques* (2nd edition, 43). HRST Books, 2009.

[10] Rennells, 123.

[4] Massey, Lorraine, with Michele Bender. *Curly Girl*. Thomas Allen & Son Limited, 14, 2010.

[9] Massey, 41.

[5] Walker, Andre. *Andre Talks Hair!* Simon & Schuster, 46, 1999.

[6] Rennells, Lauren. *Vintage Hairstyling Retro Styles with Step-by-Step Techniques* (2nd edition). HRST Books, 15, 2009.

[7] Turudich, Daniela. *1940s Hairstyling*. Streamline Press, 15, 2010.

[8] "Fated to Frizz"—*New York Times* http://www.nytimes.com/2012/10/30/science/why-does-some-hair-frizz-when-its-humid.html?_r=0/ Last Viewed February 15, 2013.

[14] Kinard, Tulani. *No Lye!* St. Martin's Press, 103, 1997.

Chapter 4—Styling Tools & Aid Questions

[1] Mayost, Eric. *Gorgeous Wedding Hairstyles: A Step-by-Step Guide to 34 Spectacular Hairstyles*. Penn Publishing Ltd., 6, 2012.

[4] Mayost, 7.

[2] Rennells, Lauren. *Vintage Hairstyling Retro Styles with Step-by-Step Techniques* (2nd edition). HRST Books, 15, 2009.

[5] Rennells, 14.

[7] Rennells, 13.

[8] Rennells, 12.

[3] "What Is 'Ionic' Technology & Why Is It Good For Your Hair?"—Larry Dunlap Hairstyling _http://www.larry-dunlaphairstyling.com/article_ionic.html_ Last Viewed February 25, 2013.

[6] "Need Help Choosing a Denman Product"— _http://www.denmanbrushus.com/acatalog/hair-brushes.html_ Last viewed February 18,2013.

Chapter 6—Chemicals and the Natural Hair

[1] Fletcher, Barry. _Why Are Black Women Losing Their Hair?_ Unity Publishers, Inc., 101, 2000.

[2] Fletcher, 99.

[3] Fletcher, 98–102.

[4] Fletcher, 100.

[5] "What is a carcinogen?"—American Cancer Society _http://www.cancer.org/Cancer/CancerCauses/OtherCarcinogens/GeneralInformationaboutCarcinogens/known-and-probable-human-carcinogens/_ Last Viewed February 24, 2013.

Chapter 7—Transitioning Away from Chemicals

[1] Massey, Lorraine, with Michele Bender. *Curly Girl*. Thomas Allen & Son Limited, 14, 2010.

Chapter 8—Shampooing, Conditioning & Hair Treatments for Transitioners

[1] Evans, Nekhena. *Hairlocking: Everything You Need to Know, African, Dreads & Nubian Locks*. A&B Publishers Group, 50, 1999.

[2] Evens, 51.

Chapter 9—General Information for Locked Hair

[1] Evans, Nekhena. *Hairlocking: Everything You Need to Know, African, Dreads & Nubian Locks*. A&B Publishers Group, 53, 1999.

[2] Bonner, Lonnice Brittenum. *Plaited Glory: For Colored Girls Who've Considered Braids, Locks, and Twists*. Three River Press, 43, 1996.

[3] Bonner, 42.

[4] Bonner, Lonnice Brittenum. *Nice Dreads*. Three River Press, 71, 2005.

[5] Bonner, Lonnice Brittenum. *Nice Dreads*. Three River Press, 88, 2005.

[6] Bonner, Lonnice Brittenum. *Nice Dreads*. Three River

Press, 89, 2005.

Chapter 10—Shampooing, Conditioning & Treatments for Locks

[1] Bonner, Lonnice Brittenum. *Nice Dreads.* Three River Press, 53, 2005.

[2] Massey, Lorraine, with Michele Bender. *Curly Girl.* Thomas Allen & Son Limited, 42, 2010.

[3] Bonner, Lonnice Brittenum. *Nice Dreads.* Three River Press, 91, 2005.

Chapter 14—Natural Hair in the Workplace

[1] Shipp, E.R. (1997). *New York Times, http://
www.nytimes.com/1987/09/23/garden/braided-
hair-style-at-issue-in-protests-over-dress-codes.
html?pagewanted=all&src=pm/* Last Viewed February 26, 2013.